R-2712-HHS

Development of a Dental Satisfaction Questionnaire for the Health Insurance Experiment

Allyson Ross Davies and John E. Ware, Jr.

April 1982

Prepared under a grant from the
U.S. Department of Health and Human Services

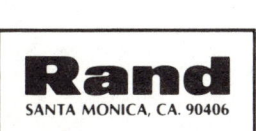

PREFACE

This report was written as part of Rand's Health Insurance Experiment, funded under a grant from the U.S. Department of Health and Human Services. It evaluates, against standard psychometric criteria, the adequacy of the measures used to assess satisfaction with dental care for adults in the experiment. The psychometric analyses use data from enrollment Medical History Questionnaires and annual Health Questionnaires in the six study sites. The information in this report is directed to those who will be using the dental care satisfaction measures in the Health Insurance Experiment's analyses, and to others who are interested in using or adapting these measures for their own research. A much-abbreviated version of this report appeared in *Social Science and Medicine,* 15A:751-760, December 1981.

The dental satisfaction measures are among several sets of measures that provide data on outcomes for experimental analyses of the effects of coinsurance and deductible rates. Several other Rand reports and report series issued as part of the Health Insurance Experiment discuss the health status outcome measures. They include:

R-1987-HEW, *Conceptualization and Measurement of Health for Adults in the Health Insurance Study,* Vols. I-VIII, multiple authors, July 1978 through December 1980.

R-2313-HEW, *Conceptualization and Measurement of Health for Children in the Health Insurance Study,* Marvin Eisen, Cathy A. Donald, John E. Ware, Jr., and Robert H. Brook, May 1980.

R-2262-HHS, *Conceptualization and Measurement of Physiologic Health for Adults,* Vols. 1-18, multiple authors, August 1980 and continuing. This set will include a volume that describes the measures of dental health status and quality of dental care used in the experimental analyses.

Additional reports from the Health Insurance Experiment that may be of interest to a dental care audience include:

R-2126-HEW, *The Methodology Used To Measure Health Care Consumption during the First Year of the Health Insurance Experiment,* Kent H. Marquis, August 1977.

R-2157-HEW, *Dental Care Demand: Point Estimates and Implications for National Health Insurance,* Willard G. Manning, Jr., and Charles E. Phelps, March 1978.

A complete list of study papers and reports issued through 1978 appears in P-6221, *Overview of Health Insurance Study Publications,* Joseph P. Newhouse and Rae W. Archibald, November 1978.

SUMMARY

Measures of dental care satisfaction will be used in the Health Insurance Experiment's (HIE) analyses as dependent variables to test hypotheses about differences in satisfaction as a function of coinsurance and deductible rates, and as covariates in studies of relationships among coinsurance rate, use of dental services, and dental health status. This report describes the development of a self-administered Dental Satisfaction Questionnaire (DSQ) for use in the HIE, and presents results of analyses designed to evaluate how well the DSQ met the goals outlined for its development and usefulness to the HIE. These goals were (1) a short but comprehensive battery of items; (2) multi-item measures of the major dental satisfaction constructs; (3) sufficient variability in scores on the measures; (4) sufficient reliability for group comparisons; and (5) valid measures. Results of our analyses indicate that the DSQ generally meets these goals; further work remains to validate the measures against additional external criteria.

The DSQ was designed for self-administration by respondents aged 14 and older and requires about 5 minutes to complete. Items refer to quality of care (both technical and interpersonal aspects), accessibility (nonfinancial and financial aspects), availability, convenience, continuity, efficacy/outcomes, general satisfaction, and pain management. These items represent all but two (practice organization, specific features of treatment) of the dimensions of dental care satisfaction identified in our literature review. Given the interest in assessing attitudes toward interpersonal aspects of dental care that is apparent in the literature, this construct is underrepresented in the DSQ, and we offer several suggestions for the improvement of this measure.

Scaling analyses resulted in construction of nine dental satisfaction measures. Five multi-item subscales assess attitudes toward Access, Availability/Convenience, Cost, Pain Management, and Quality; two single-item measures assess Continuity and General Satisfaction; an Access Total scale aggregates the access-related subscales; and the overall Dental Satisfaction Index combines all the single- and multi-item subscales. Tests of item discriminant validity and factor analyses support the hypothesized item groupings and indicate the multidimensional nature of the dental satisfaction concept.

Variability appears to be adequate for testing hypotheses about differences in group means, and for correlational studies with these measures. Analyses indicate that reliability estimates for the multi-item scales meet or exceed 0.50 in all sites with only one exception; reliability estimates for the overall Index approach 0.90. Thus, scores on these measures will prove reliable enough for group comparisons, their intended use in HIE experimental analyses.

Content analyses of the DSQ items indicate that each one appears to assess the intended dental satisfaction construct (face validity), and that they represent most of the major satisfaction dimensions identified in the literature (content validity). Empirical evidence of validity included multitrait and factor analytic scaling studies, which supported the multidimensional conceptualization of dental satisfaction and the discriminant validity of the items. Discriminant validity of the scales as measures of distinct but related satisfaction dimensions was supported by analyses of scale intercorrelations and of correlations between dental and medical satisfaction measures.

These lines of evidence support the validity of the measures, and argue for the separate scoring and interpretation of DSQ subscales. Further validity studies, not possible until additional HIE data become available, will focus on the validity of DSQ measures as indicators of differences in the structure and process of dental care, and as predictors of dental health-related behaviors.

We also studied several methodological issues, including the effect of different types of response sets (acquiescent, opposition, social desirability) and the effect of questionnaire placement on DSQ scale scores.

In conclusion, the available evidence supports the usefulness of the DSQ to HIE experimental analyses. The DSQ yields variable and reliable scores for each of the major dental satisfaction constructs in general populations. Improvements should be made in the representativeness of the battery with respect to interpersonal aspects of dental care. The available evidence is also consistent with the interpretation of scores as indicators of the intended dental satisfaction constructs, although more work remains to be done in this area. Further work is also needed to fully clarify the distinction between dental and medical care satisfaction. The results support use of the DSQ in general population studies that focus on patients' viewpoints regarding dental care; to support that use, the volume includes scale scoring rules and suggests modifications and areas for future research on the dental satisfaction concept.

ACKNOWLEDGMENTS

We would like to acknowledge the comments made on an earlier draft of this report by Marilyn Bergner, University of Washington School of Public Health; Howard Bailit, University of Connecticut School of Dental Medicine; and our Rand colleague, Joseph P. Newhouse. To William A. Ayer at the American Dental Association's Health Foundation and Lois K. Cohen at the National Institute of Dental Research go our thanks for their interest in seeing the journal version of this report published.

CONTENTS

PREFACE iii
SUMMARY v
ACKNOWLEDGMENTS vii
TABLES xi

Section

I. INTRODUCTION 1
    Background 1
    Goals for Development of the Dental Satisfaction Questionnaire 1
    Organization of the Report 2

II. LITERATURE REVIEW 3
    Uses of Dental Satisfaction Measures 3
    Dimensions of Dental Care Satisfaction 4
        Content Analyses 4
        Empirical Analyses 13
    Score Variability 14
    Reliability and Validity 14
    Sociodemographic Correlates of Dental Satisfaction 16
    Summary 16

III. DEVELOPMENT OF THE HIE DENTAL SATISFACTION
      QUESTIONNAIRE 18
    Item Development 18
    Administration of the DSQ in the Health Insurance Experiment 18

IV. METHODS 20
    Data-Gathering Methods 20
    Sample Characteristics 20
    Analysis Plan 22
    Methods of Analysis 22
        Item Scoring 22
        Scale Construction Methods 23
        Reliability 24
        Validity of Dental Satisfaction Measures 25
        Methods of Studying Response Sets 25

V. RESULTS 27
    Descriptive Statistics: Items 27
    Missing Data 27
    Scale Construction 28
        Analysis of Item Internal Consistency 29
        Analysis of Item Discriminant Validity 31
        Principal Components Analysis 32

	Scoring the DSQ Scales	35
	Descriptive Statistics: Dental Satisfaction Scales	35
	Reliability of Scale Scores	35
	Effect of Questionnaire Placement	37
	Validity of Scale Scores	37
	Face and Content Validity	38
	Construct Validity	39
	Threats to Validity: Response Sets	44
	Differences between Dental and Medical Care Satisfaction	46
	Sociodemographic Correlates of Dental Satisfaction Measures	47
VI.	DISCUSSION	48
	Comprehensiveness of Measurement	48
	Dimensionality of Patient Satisfaction	49
	Studying the Dimensions	49
	Scoring the Dimensions	50
	Score Variability	51
	Reliability	52
	Validity	53
	Comparing Dental and Medical Care Satisfaction	55
	Group Differences in Dental Satisfaction	56
	Conclusions	56

Appendix

A.	DENTAL SATISFACTION QUESTIONNAIRE	59
B.	DSQ ITEM AND SCALE SCORING RULES	63
C.	ITEMS USED TO MEASURE RESPONSE SET AND RESPONSE SET SCORING RULES	65
D.	SUPPORTING TABLES	67
E.	RECOMMENDED ADDITIONS TO DENTAL SATISFACTION QUESTIONNAIRE TO MEASURE INTERPERSONAL ASPECTS OF DENTAL CARE	91

REFERENCES 93

TABLES

1. Content of Published Dental Satisfaction Measures 1
2. Abbreviated Item Content, Direction of Wording, and Content Category, Dental Satisfaction Items 19
3. Summary of Sample Characteristics for Analyses of Dental Satisfaction Measures 21
4. Means and Standard Deviations, Dental Satisfaction Items, All Sites Combined . 28
5. Correlations between DSQ Items and Hypothesized Subscales, All Sites Combined 29
6. Correlations between DSQ Items and Hypothesized Global Scales, All Sites Combined 30
7. Number of Item Discriminant Validity Successes for Dental Satisfaction Scales, by Site and All Sites Combined 31
8. Homogeneity Estimates, Dental Satisfaction Scales, All Sites Combined 32
9. Correlations between DSQ Items and Four Rotated Principal Components, All Sites Combined 34
10. Means, Standard Deviations, and Scale Midpoints, Dental Satisfaction Measures, All Sites Combined 36
11. Reliability Estimates for Dental Satisfaction Scales, All Sites Combined and by Site 36
12. Effect of Questionnaire Placement on Mean Dental Satisfaction Scores, Two Sites 38
13. Effect of Questionnaire Placement on Dental Satisfaction Score Reliability, Multi-Item Measures, Two Sites 39
14. Correlations among Dental Satisfaction Scales 40
15. Unstandardized and Standardized Regression Coefficients for Prediction of General Satisfaction with Dental Care, by Dimensions of Dental Satisfaction ... 41
16. Correlations between Dental and Medical Satisfaction Items, All Sites Combined 43
17. First Two Rotated Principal Components from Matched Dental and Medical Care Satisfaction Items 44
18. Correlations between Social Desirability Response Set and Dental Satisfaction Measures and Sociodemographic Variables 45
19. Comparison between Ratings of Dental and Medical Care on Matched Questionnaire Items 46
20. Sociodemographic Correlates of Dental Satisfaction Measures, All Sites Combined 47
B.1. Scoring Rules for Items/Scoring Rules for Scales, 19-Item Dental Satisfaction Questionnaire 63
B.2. Scoring Rules for Items/Scoring Rules for Scales, 14-Item Dental Satisfaction Questionnaire 64
C.1. Matched Pairs Used To Score Acquiescent and Opposition Response Sets 65
C.2. Items and Scoring Rules for Social Desirability Response Set Measure 66

D.1.	Frequency Distributions for Responses to DSQ Items, by Site and All Sites Combined	67
D.2.	Means and Standard Deviations, DSQ Items, by Site	70
D.3.	Correlations between DSQ Items and Hypothesized Subscales, Dayton	71
D.4.	Correlations between DSQ Items and Hypothesized Subscales, Seattle	72
D.5.	Correlations between DSQ Items and Hypothesized Subscales, Massachusetts	73
D.6.	Correlations between DSQ Items and Hypothesized Subscales, South Carolina	74
D.7.	Correlations between DSQ Items and Hypothesized Global Scales, Dayton	75
D.8.	Correlations between DSQ Items and Hypothesized Global Scales, Seattle	76
D.9.	Correlations between DSQ Items and Hypothesized Global Scales, Massachusetts	77
D.10.	Correlations between DSQ Items and Hypothesized Global Scales, South Carolina	78
D.11.	Cumulative Percent of Variance Explained in DSQ Items by One to Six Principal Components, All Sites Combined	79
D.12.	Means, Standard Deviations, and Scale Midpoints, Dental Satisfaction Measures, by Site	80
D.13.	Frequency Distributions for Access Scale, by Site	81
D.14.	Frequency Distributions for Availability/Convenience Scale, by Site	81
D.15.	Frequency Distributions for Cost Scale, by Site	82
D.16.	Frequency Distributions for Pain Scale, by Site	82
D.17.	Frequency Distributions for Quality Scale, by Site	83
D.18.	Frequency Distributions for Access Total Scale, by Site	84
D.19.	Frequency Distributions for Dental Satisfaction Index, by Site	85
D.20.	Comparison between Ratings of Dental and Medical Care on Matched Questionnaire Items, Dayton	87
D.21.	Comparison between Ratings of Dental and Medical Care on Matched Questionnaire Items, Seattle	88
D.22.	Comparison between Ratings of Dental and Medical Care on Matched Questionnaire Items, Massachusetts	89
D.23.	Comparison between Ratings of Dental and Medical Care on Matched Questionnaire Items, South Carolina	90

I. INTRODUCTION

BACKGROUND

The Health Insurance Experiment (HIE) is a social experiment designed to evaluate the effects of differences in health care financing (differing coinsurance and deductible rates) on use of services, health status, quality of care, and patient satisfaction.[1] Coverage of virtually all dental services but preventive orthodontia is included in the comprehensive benefits package provided to all enrollees. Patient satisfaction with dental care is thus an important outcome for analysis in the study, and development of a dental satisfaction measure a necessary prerequisite to data collection and analyses of experimental data. Dental care satisfaction scores will be used in HIE analyses as dependent variables to test hypotheses about differences in patient satisfaction as a function of coinsurance, and as covariates to study relationships among coinsurance rate, use of dental services, and dental health status.

This report describes the development of the Dental Satisfaction Questionnaire (DSQ) for use in the HIE, and presents analyses of its scoring, reliability, and validity based on data from HIE enrollees in the six study sites.[2] The information presented here should be useful to those who are interested in knowing how dental satisfaction is measured in the HIE. It will also be useful to those who are involved in selecting and developing measures to assess satisfaction as an outcome measure in evaluations of dental care or as a predictor in studies of patient behavior.

GOALS FOR DEVELOPMENT OF THE DENTAL SATISFACTION QUESTIONNAIRE

Five goals guided development of the DSQ, a self-administered battery of items to measure dental care satisfaction. First, we wanted a comprehensive battery, including items that assess all major dimensions of satisfaction and dissatisfaction with dental care providers and services, and that represent positive and negative attitudes on each dimension. Within this guideline, the battery had to be short—some 15 to 20 items, requiring four to five minutes to complete—because it is included in HIE questionnaires along with several hundred health-related items. Second, because levels of satisfaction may differ depending on the dimension of care considered, we wanted to construct a multi-item measure of each major dimension as well as an overall index that aggregates across the dimensions. Third, we sought sufficient variability in score distributions to permit finer distinctions in sentiment than simply that respondents had generally favorable or unfavorable attitudes; for example, distinguishing differences in satisfaction among those with generally favorable sentiments. Fourth, we required scores that would prove reliable enough for making group comparisons, their chief use

---

[1]Background information and a description of the Health Insurance Experiment's design and the experimental health insurance plans appear in Newhouse (1974) and Ware, Brook, Davies-Avery, et al. (1980, Sec. II).

[2]Dayton, Ohio; Seattle, Washington; Franklin County and Fitchburg, Massachusetts; Georgetown County and Charleston, South Carolina. For all enrollees but those adults in Dayton on the nonfree plans, dental services were covered from the outset of the experiment; Dayton nonfree plan enrollees were covered for dental services after their first year of participation. This report deals with dental satisfaction measures developed for use with enrollees aged 14 and older.

in HIE hypothesis-testing. Finally, we needed valid measures, on which scores could confidently be interpreted as reflecting satisfaction with dental care services and providers rather than some other concept.

ORGANIZATION OF THE REPORT

Section II presents a literature review that identifies the major dimensions of satisfaction with dental care and summarizes available information about the reliability and validity of earlier dental satisfaction measures for comparison with HIE results. Section III describes development of items for the HIE dental satisfaction battery, and Sec. IV, our data-gathering methods, sample characteristics, analysis plan, and analytic procedures. Section V presents results from our studies to construct dental satisfaction scales and from the reliability and validity analyses. That section also includes a comparison of enrollees' attitudes about their dental and medical care, and data on the sociodemographic correlates of the dental satisfaction measures. In Sec. VI, we discuss these results in terms of the goals we outlined earlier for the DSQ, and offer conclusions and recommendations concerning the usefulness of the measures for the HIE and for other research on dental satisfaction. The DSQ and its scoring rules appear in the appendixes, as do the supporting tables.

II. LITERATURE REVIEW

Our search for literature published during the past decade or so on dental care satisfaction yielded some 25 empirical articles. Our review of these publications examines the uses of dental satisfaction measures, the dimensions of satisfaction revealed in item content and through empirical studies of their relationships, and available evidence about the variability, reliability, and validity of satisfaction scores.

Not all investigators use the term "satisfaction" to refer to their measures; some apply the term "attitude" and others, "perception." What is common to all the measures we discuss is that they ask for an *evaluation* of some aspect of dental providers and services, or imply an evaluative assessment on the respondent's part. Some measures that used the "satisfaction" label were actually measures of satisfaction with dental health status, attitudes about dental health, and attitudes regarding the dental profession and use of auxiliary personnel. We did not consider these measures appropriate for inclusion in our review.

USES OF DENTAL SATISFACTION MEASURES

Dental care satisfaction measures have most commonly been fielded to study attitudes toward dental care and use of dental services, including care-seeking behavior. Several investigators studied attitudes toward dentists and dental care in the United States (Kriesberg and Treiman, 1962; McKeithen, 1966; Collett, 1969; Jenny et al., 1973); others examined these attitudes among populations in Great Britain (Richards et al., 1965; Scarrott, 1969). Several studies focused on the dental attitudes and behaviors of college students, particularly in relation to nonuse of services (Fanning and Leppard, 1973; Belok, 1977; Blum and Tuthill, 1977; Stacey, Slome, and Musgrave, 1978). Others who examined the relationships between attitudes and use or nonuse of dental care include Bene, Novasky, and Geldart (1974) and Murray and Wiese (1975). The relationships between individual characteristics and attitudes toward care was the subject of a study by Strauss (1976). Others have used dental satisfaction measures to evaluate care, including the quality of care provided to persons eligible for pre-paid dental care benefits (Bailit and Raskin, 1978), and the dentist-patient relationship (Biro and Hewson, 1976). Two studies were done specifically to develop dental care satisfaction measures (Koslowsky, Bailit, and Valluzzo, 1974; Hengst and Roghmann, 1978); another developed a new dental care satisfaction measure during the research (Murray and Wiese, 1975).

Information about questionnaire administration methods was mentioned in 17 of the studies. Self-administration, usually with mail-out and mail-back procedures, was used in seven studies; another seven used interviewers. Three sets of investigators used both techniques, each for different subsamples in their study populations. Response rates were reported for 12 studies, and ranged from 42.8 percent to 96 percent with a median of 63.2 percent.

Virtually all studies relied on cross-sectional designs. Most studies that linked satisfaction to use of services and other dental health-related behavior obtained information about use from the respondents. Murray and Wiese (1975) did a retrospective study of use and satisfaction, tracking use of services through dental records and appointment logs and then administering satisfaction questionnaires to the user and nonuser samples they had identified. Although some investigators "predicted" use with satisfaction scores, their conclusions were based on the questionable assumption that satisfaction scores obtained *after* experiences with dental care services and providers were not affected by those experiences.

DIMENSIONS OF DENTAL CARE SATISFACTION

The dimensions of dental care satisfaction comprise distinguishable features of care that influence attitudes toward providers and services. Investigators have used several different techniques to reveal these dimensions. Some asked open-ended questions about the things people liked and disliked most about dentists and dental care, or about the best and worst attributes of dentists and dental care (Kriesberg and Treiman, 1962; McKeithen, 1966) and content-analyzed the responses. Others asked whether patients were satisfied or dissatisfied and their reasons for holding that attitude (Jenny et al., 1973; Murray and Wiese, 1975) and similarly examined their content. Several investigators fielded a wide range of satisfaction items found in literature reviews or developed for a particular study and studied empirically the common constructs underlying the various items (Koslowsky, Bailit, and Valluzzo, 1974; Murray and Wiese, 1975; Hengst and Roghmann, 1978).

Because not all investigators used the same labels to refer to measures with similar content, the similarity of dimensions and item content was not always apparent. To reduce the confusion, we proposed a "taxonomy" of dental satisfaction like the one we have used to study measures of satisfaction with medical care (Ware, Davies-Avery, and Stewart, 1978). Those dimensions and a brief definition of each are given below:

- Technical: aspects of care related to the process of diagnosis and treatment.
- Interpersonal: aspects of care related to the provider's style or manner of dealing with the patient as an individual (sometimes labeled art of care).
- Accessibility/Availability: process of arranging for and getting to care, including presence and convenience of services.
- Financial access: financial aspects of arranging for care, including cost of care.
- Efficacy/Outcomes: effectiveness of care and results of treatment.
- Continuity: sameness of dental care provider.
- Facilities: office environment and atmosphere.
- General: attitudes about overall care, not referring to a specific dimension.

Content Analyses

Several investigators analyzed the content of responses to open-ended questions regarding dental care and providers to categorize the major dimensions of dental satisfaction or attitudes. Kriesberg and Treiman (1962) studied the content of responses to open-ended questions that asked about the most- and least-liked aspects of dentists; respondents were 1,862 adults participating in a National Opinion Research Center survey. More than 90 percent of the respondents commented on favorable characteristics, while only 28 to 33 percent made unfavorable comments about characteristics of their regular dentist or the last dentist they had seen.

Similar dimensions emerged from both the favorable and unfavorable responses. Comments on the things liked most about regular dentists indicated that major dimensions were quality of care (technical and interpersonal aspects about equal, with some 65 percent of respondents commenting on this characteristic), office environment/facilities (about 40 percent), pain management (about 20 percent), financial aspects (about 15 percent), accessibility (about 10 percent), and other (about 10 percent).[1] Comments about disliked aspects of dental care mentioned office environment/facilities and accessibility about as frequently (7 percent each), financial aspects (about 5 percent), quality (technical and interpersonal aspects equal at about 3 percent), pain management (another 3 percent), and other (some 10 percent).

McKeithen (1966) noted similar findings in content analyses of responses to open-ended items asking for descriptions of the best and worst imaginable dentists; responding were 400 adult members of a prepaid group practice in Washington, D.C. Her study also indicated that respondents were more apt to describe favorable than unfavorable characteristics of dentists. Although we could not determine the percentage of respondents commenting about each dimension from her published data, the dimensions revealed by the comments included technical and interpersonal aspects of quality, financial access, pain management, facilities, availability, and organization of practice.

Jenny et al. (1973) asked parents who reported that they were satisfied with their child's dentist to describe the reasons for their satisfaction; they surveyed the parents of 838 white fourth graders in an unnamed large city. Some 90 percent of parents thought their child's care was good and were satisfied with the dentist. No representative content was given, so we could not determine whether they classified item content in the same categories that we would have. The dimensions reported by Jenny et al., along with the labels from our taxonomy that appear to best represent the labels they used, include: interpersonal (relationship with children, 37 percent of parents; personal characteristics of dentist, 34 percent); technical (professional competence, 52 percent; explanations, 9 percent; reputation, 4 percent; office procedures/periodic recall, 3 percent; preventive procedures, 2 percent); convenience of location (12 percent); financial access (9 percent); accessibility in emergency (3 percent).

In addition to fielding a multi-item satisfaction battery, Murray and Wiese (1975) asked respondents an open-ended question about the reasons for their satisfaction and dissatisfaction with care; respondents were 40 patients at a neighborhood health center's dental clinic in Lexington, Kentucky. As in the previously discussed studies, more people mentioned reasons for satisfaction than dissatisfaction. The dimensions revealed in the favorable comments include technical aspects (about 58 percent of respondents commenting), interpersonal aspects (about 37 percent), and financial aspects (5 percent). Reasons for dissatisfaction revealed dimensions of accessibility (40 percent) and technical aspects of care (30 percent).

Using our proposed taxonomy, we did a content analysis of all the single- and multi-item measures that we found in the literature; the analysis appears in Table 1. Entries in the table represent abbreviated item content from the measures we analyzed or abbreviated responses from the open-ended comments analyzed by others and reported in their studies. The categories are listed roughly in order of the frequency of their measurement; within each category, items or responses with similar content are grouped together.[2] As we categorized items, we noted two groupings that had not appeared in our proposed taxonomy, and thus expanded it to include "organization of practice" and "specific features of treatment." A couple of items whose content did not appear similar to any others were categorized as "other."

Our analysis indicates that, across studies, technical aspects of dental care and providers

---

[1] Percentages add to more than 100 because respondents commented on more than one characteristic.
[2] Because Jenny et al. (1973) reported only major categories and did not include representative content, no entries from their study appear in the table.

Table 1

CONTENT OF PUBLISHED DENTAL SATISFACTION MEASURES

Content Category	Investigators
TECHNICAL QUALITY	
dentist provides good to excellent dental care	Bailit and Raskin (1978)
does good work	Kriesberg and Treiman (1962)
does poor work	Kriesberg and Treiman (1962)
quality of work by dentist	Murray and Wiese (1975)
work carelessly done	Collett (1969)
dental qualifications	Scarrott (1969)
modern, progressive	McKeithen (1966)
dentist keeps up with latest techniques	Koslowsky et al. (1974)
old fashioned, doesn't keep up with advances	Kriesberg and Treiman (1962)
uses latest equipment, techniques	McKeithen (1966)
competent	Kriesberg and Treiman (1962)
well-trained	McKeithen (1966); Kriesberg and Treiman (1962)
incompetent	Kriesberg and Treiman (1962)
technically competent	McKeithen (1966)
dentist's perceived competency	Murray and Wiese (1975)
competent personnel	Murray and Wiese (1975)
incompetent auxiliary personnel	Murray and Wiese (1975)
not well-trained	McKeithen (1966); Kriesberg and Treiman (1962)
skillful	McKeithen (1966); Kriesberg and Treiman (1962)
well-informed, experienced	McKeithen (1966)
modern equipment	Scarrott (1969)
modern office, well-equipped	Kriesberg and Treiman (1962)
good equipment	Kriesberg and Treiman (1962)
old, poor, inadequate equipment	Kriesberg and Treiman (1962)

Table 1—continued

Content Category	Investigators
TECHNICAL QUALITY, cont'd.	
confidence in dentist	Biro and Hewson (1976)
confidence in the care of my dentist	Koslowsky et al. (1974)
inspires trust	McKeithen (1966)
careful, conscientious	McKeithen (1966)
dentist always thorough in his examination	Koslowsky et al. (1974)
thorough, careful	Kriesberg and Treiman (1962)
not thorough enough	Kriesberg and Treiman (1962)
information about treatment	Scarrott (1969)
explains what work needs to be done	McKeithen (1966)
maps out program	McKeithen (1966)
dentists clearly explain what is wrong before giving you treatment	Hengst and Roghmann (1978)
dentist answers my questions fully	Koslowsky et al. (1974)
answers questions	McKeithen (1966); Kriesberg and Treiman (1962)
doesn't answer questions	Kriesberg and Treiman (1962)
does unnecessary work	Collett (1969)
recommends unnecessary work	Kriesberg and Treiman (1962)
does only necessary work	McKeithen (1966)
prevention orientation	Murray and Wiese (1975)
stresses preventive aspects	McKeithen (1966)
provides dental education	McKeithen (1966)
dentists teach patients how to prevent dental problems	Hengst and Roghmann (1978)
dentist careless with instruments	Koslowsky et al. (1974)
calls in specialists when needed	McKeithen (1966)
dentist's reputation	Murray and Wiese (1975)
tries to save teeth	McKeithen (1966)
dentist's knowledge of patient's teeth	Scarrott (1969)
knows case	Kriesberg and Treiman (1962)

Table 1—continued

Content Category	Investigators
INTERPERSONAL ASPECTS	
patient's concept of dentist's attitude	Biro and Hewson (1976)
dentist's attitude or manner	Fanning and Leppard (1973)
sympathetic attitude	Scarrott (1969)
understanding, sympathetic	McKeithen (1966)
dentist sympathetic to my problems	Koslowsky et al. (1974)
most dentists take a real interest in their patients	Hengst and Roghmann (1978)
not impersonal	McKeithen (1966)
impersonal treatment	Scarrott (1969)
takes personal interest	Kriesberg and Treiman (1962)
not friendly enough	Kriesberg and Treiman (1962)
dentist does not care about me as a person	Koslowsky et al. (1974)
many dentists treat the disease but have no feeling for the patient	Hengst and Roghmann (1978)
perceived empathy of the dentist	Murray and Wiese (1975)
dentist friendly	Koslowsky et al. (1974)
pleasant, friendly, social	McKeithen (1966)
dentists should be a little more friendly than they are	Hengst and Roghmann (1978)
dentist not warm and friendly	Collett (1969)
dentist explains things to me	Koslowsky et al. (1974)
explains what he is doing	McKeithen (1966)
takes time to explain condition	Kriesberg and Treiman (1962)
doesn't take time to explain things	Kriesberg and Treiman (1962)
reassures patient	McKeithen (1966)
puts patient at ease	Kriesberg and Treiman (1962)
sees to patient's comfort	McKeithen (1966)
polite, courteous	Kriesberg and Treiman (1962)
too authoritarian, interfering	Kriesberg and Treiman (1962)

Table 1—continued

Content Category	Investigators
INTERPERSONAL ASPECTS, cont'd.	
dentist has good to excellent personal manners	Bailit and Raskin (1978)
personal friend, known for a long time	Kriesberg and Treiman (1962)
dentist has poor personality	Collett (1969)
habits, mannerisms, personal life	Kriesberg and Treiman (1962)
equalitarian	Kriesberg and Treiman (1962)
listens	Kriesberg and Treiman (1962)
kind	Kriesberg and Treiman (1962)
good with children	Kriesberg and Treiman (1962)
sure of himself, self-confident	Kriesberg and Treiman (1962)
dentist's self-image	Murray and Wiese (1975)
serious, business-like	Kriesberg and Treiman (1962)
jovial, good-natured, happy, not stuffy	Kriesberg and Treiman (1962)
too serious, too quiet	Kriesberg and Treiman (1962)
pleasant assistants, nurse	Kriesberg and Treiman (1962)
reception, treatment by auxiliary personnel	Murray and Wiese (1975)
assistants, nurse not pleasant	Kriesberg and Treiman (1962)
ACCESSIBILITY/CONVENIENCE	
seldom have problems scheduling convenient dental appointment	Bailit and Raskin (1978)
readily available appointments	Scarrott (1969)
reasonable time to wait for an appointment in nonemergency	Bene et al. (1974)
difficult to get appointment	Blum and Tuthill (1977)
no difficulty making an appointment	Koslowsky et al. (1974)
easy to get appointment	Kriesberg and Treiman (1962)
don't need an appointment	Kriesberg and Treiman (1962)
appointments scheduled too far in advance	Murray and Wiese (1975)

Table 1—continued

Content Category	Investigators
ACCESSIBILITY/CONVENIENCE, cont'd.	
in an emergency, you can always get a dentist	Hengst and Roghmann (1978)
not always available	Kriesberg and Treiman (1962)
dentist easy to reach on evenings, weekends, and holidays	Koslowsky et al. (1974)
no problem with transportation to dental office	Bailit and Raskin (1978)
accessibility of dentist's office	Bene et al. (1974)
dentists try to have their offices and clinics in convenient locations	Hengst and Roghmann (1978)
office not conveniently located, too far away	Kriesberg and Treiman (1962)
once get into dentist's chair, treatment begins at once	Koslowsky et al. (1974)
doesn't keep you waiting	Kriesberg and Treiman (1962)
keeps appointment on time	McKeithen (1966)
dentists do not care how long the patients have to wait	Hengst and Roghmann (1978)
keeps you waiting	Kriesberg and Treiman (1962)
waiting time for treatment	Murray and Wiese (1975)
FINANCIAL ASPECTS	
dental costs in general	Bene et al. (1974)
costs of dental services relative to costs of other services	Bene et al. (1974)
expense of care	Blum and Tuthill (1977)
fees too high	Collett (1969); Kriesberg and Treiman (1962)
reasonable rates	McKeithen (1966)
cost of care	Murray and Wiese (1975)
fees are reasonable, not expensive	Kriesberg and Treiman (1962)
dentist discusses costs of treatment before proceeding	Koslowsky et al. (1974)

Table 1—continued

Content Category	Investigators
FINANCIAL ASPECTS, cont'd.	
dentist sensitive to possible financial problems when he sets fees	Koslowsky et al. (1974)
tries to keep dental costs down	Kriesberg and Treiman (1962)
patient about his bill	Kriesberg and Treiman (1962)
unreasonable about bill	Kriesberg and Treiman (1962)
not mercenary	Kriesberg and Treiman (1962); McKeithen (1966)
mercenary	Kriesberg and Treiman (1962)
dentist too concerned with money	Koslowsky et al. (1974)
PAIN MANAGEMENT/DENTAL PAIN	
many dentists do not care whether or not they hurt you	Hengst and Roghmann (1978)
gentle, tries not to hurt patient	Kriesberg and Treiman (1962)
talks to keep mind off pain	McKeithen (1966)
dentist's concern for relieving pain	Murray and Wiese (1975)
painless, avoids pain, tries not to hurt	McKeithen (1966)
causes pain, hurts patient	Kriesberg and Treiman (1962)
rough, doesn't care if he hurts patient	Kriesberg and Treiman (1962)
sympathetic toward pain	McKeithen (1966)
causes very little pain because of skill, use of drugs, etc.	Kriesberg and Treiman (1962)
fear of pain in general	Fanning and Leppard (1973)
fear of pain from drill	Fanning and Leppard (1973)
dislike dental pain	Scarrott (1969)
pain	Murray and Wiese (1975)
GENERAL SATISFACTION	
satisfaction with past dental care	Belok (1977)
patient's attitude toward dentist	Biro and Hewson (1976)

Table 1—continued

Content Category	Investigators
GENERAL SATISFACTION, cont'd.	
satisfaction with care in recent dental emergency	Bene et al. (1974)
satisfaction with dental treatment	Richards et al. (1965)
satisfaction with treatment	Stacey, Slome, and Musgrave (1978)
patients receive nothing but the best of care from their dentists	Hengst and Roghmann (1978)
ORGANIZATION OF PRACTICE	
tries to treat too many patients at once	Kriesberg and Treiman (1962)
patients spend as much time as necessary with each patient	Hengst and Roghmann (1978)
does not rush or push patients around	McKeithen (1966)
concentrates on one patient at a time	McKeithen (1966)
devotes sufficient time to problem	Koslowsky et al. (1974)
SPECIFIC FEATURES OF TREATMENT	
dislike injections	Scarrott (1969)
fear of injections	Fanning and Leppard (1973)
dislike sound or feel of drill	Scarrott (1969); Fanning and Leppard (1973)
dislike treatment	Fanning and Leppard (1973)
initial probing	Scarrott (1969)
sight of equipment	Scarrott (1969)
EFFICACY/OUTCOMES	
dentist not able to relieve symptoms	Koslowsky et al. (1974)
when a dentist gets through with you, you are likely to feel worse than before	Hengst and Roghmann (1978)
CONTINUITY	
dislike changes in dentist	Scarrott (1969)

Table 1—continued

Content Category	Investigators
OTHER	
fear of dentist	Blum and Tuthill (1977)
demographic attributes, age, sex, ethnicity	Kriesberg and Treiman (1962)

is the most commonly measured dimension. Those aspects include overall quality of care, up-to-date techniques, competence of dentist and personnel, modern equipment, confidence in dentist, thoroughness, explanations and answering questions, and doing necessary work.

Interpersonal aspects of care is the second most commonly measured dimension. This dimension refers to the dentist's attitude in general, sympathetic approach, personal treatment, friendliness, reassurance, personality, and other items related to the way the dentist treats the patient personally.

Accessibility/convenience is the third most common dimension across the studies. The items in this group refer to ease of making appointments, availability of care, office location, and office waiting time. The financial access dimension captures such aspects of care as fees and payment mechanisms; a few items refer to perceived attitude of the dentist toward money. Items in the next most commonly measured dimension concern the dentist's handling of treatment-related pain and fear or pain associated with treatment. General satisfaction items were used in many studies; these items asked about attitudes in general, rather than identifying any particular aspect of care. Less frequently measured, but distinct from the preceding dimensions on the basis of content, were the dimensions of practice organization, specific features of treatment, efficacy/outcomes, and continuity.

Empirical Analyses

Classifying items by similarity of content provides an excellent first-cut at identifying the important dimensions of patient satisfaction. Empirical analyses of relationships among items are also necessary to test the appropriateness of such items groupings. Factor analytic and other scaling techniques identify items that share measured variance and reveal the underlying dimensions of dental care satisfaction. Results of the three empirical analyses that we found are consistent with the view that dental care satisfaction is a multidimensional concept. With one exception, the content of these dimensions was similar across the studies.

Koslowsky, Bailit, and Valluzzo (1974) used (unspecified) empirical techniques to identify four dimensions in the 20-item short-form of their questionnaire. They labeled these dimensions "technical competence," "personality," "organization of office," and "financial consideration." Items in the technical competence grouping refer to technical aspects of quality, symptom relief, and pain management. Those in the personality grouping include interpersonal aspects of care and information-giving. Organization of office includes items assessing convenience and accessibility of services, as well as office environment and helpfulness of nonprofessional personnel. Financial consideration items pertain to fee collection and discussion of fees before treatment.

Factor analyses of 15 items fielded by Murray and Wiese (1975) revealed three dimensions that they termed "economics," "convenience," and "quality." Our content analysis indicates that items in the economics grouping refer to financial access. Their convenience group appeared confounded because it included items related to art of care and management of pain as well as to availability/convenience of services. Their quality group included both interpersonal and technical aspects of quality.

Hengst and Roghmann (1978) adapted items for their dental satisfaction questionnaire from the medical care satisfaction battery developed by Hulka and her colleagues (Hulka et al., 1970; Zyzanski, Hulka, and Cassel, 1974), which yields measures of the provider's personal qualities, professional/technical competence, and cost/convenience of care. In multidimensional scaling studies of their final 12-item battery, Hengst and Roghmann (1978) identified two dimensions that they termed "latent hostility" and "general glorification of health professionals": these included negatively and positively worded statements, respectively. Within each dimension, items referred to interpersonal and technical aspects of care as well as access to dental care.

Thus, the content of the multi-item measures of dental care satisfaction yielded fairly similar dimensions, with the exception of Hengst and Roghmann's (1978) measure. These dimensions included technical aspects, interpersonal aspects, and access (financial or nonfinancial). These dimensions were also the most commonly assessed constructs across all measures we reviewed, single- and multi-item.

SCORE VARIABILITY

Reported mean scores on the satisfaction scales were on the side of the scale midpoints indicating more favorable sentiments. Murray and Wiese (1975) reported a mean of 59 on a scale ranging from 26 to 75. Scores were thus negatively skewed, with the mean two-thirds of the way to the highest possible score. They reported no standard deviation for an overall measure in their study sample of 40 neighborhood health center participants. Koslowsky, Bailit, and Valluzzo (1974) noted that item scores were skewed and on the favorable side of the response midpoint, as were scores on their overall scale; they reported a mean of 87.30 and standard deviation of 9.1 on a 20-item scale self-administered by 428 private dental patients. Scores in their scale could range from 20 to 100; thus, observed scores were substantially and negatively skewed, with the mean about five-sixths of the way to the highest possible score.

RELIABILITY AND VALIDITY

Underlying any interpretation of satisfaction data is the assumption that the questionnaires reliably and validly measure patient satisfaction with dental care. With the exception of studies by Koslowsky, Bailit, and Valluzzo (1974) and by Hengst and Roghmann (1978) that focused specifically on developing multi-item dental satisfaction measures, very few investigators considered the reliability of the data they analyzed. Our review identified no studies of single-item dental satisfaction measures, which are by far the most commonly fielded, that included information about reliability and validity. Only two of the three studies (Koslowsky, Bailit, and Valluzzo, 1974; Murray and Wiese, 1975; Hengst and Roghmann, 1978) that combined questionnaire items into multi-item scales reported reliability data. Koslowsky, Bailit, and Valluzzo reported an internal-consistency reliability estimate of 0.89 for the overall score constructed from their final 20-item questionnaire. Hengst and Roghmann compared Thurstone (1929) and Likert (1932) scaling of a 20-item version of their battery, and estimated internal-consistency reliabilities of 0.79 and 0.83, respectively. They did not report reliability estimates for the dimensions they obtained in multidimensional scaling studies of their final 12-item battery.

Although none of the investigators explicitly addressed measurement validity, several reported correlational data that provide information about the meaning of scores on their satisfaction measures. A common hypothesis holds that use of services will vary as a function of satisfaction (Richards, 1971; Murray and Wiese, 1975; Ware, Davies-Avery, and Stewart, 1978). Although the data were from cross-sectional studies that probably yield biased validity coefficients, several studies reported data consistent with this hypothesis. Murray and Wiese found that the more satisfied patients kept appointments. They also examined an alternative explanation for their findings; namely, that differences in the amount of exposure to dental care could predispose patients to be more or less satisfied. Controlling for exposure to care (high, medium, or low proportion of appointments kept), Murray and Wiese found no significant differences between these groups in overall satisfaction. Because of their small sample size (N = 40), however, problems in precision very likely affected their test of the alternative hypothesis and made its acceptance more likely.

Bailit and Raskin (1978) found that users were more satisfied in general and with interpersonal care than were recent nonusers; both groups had similar (and somewhat less favorable) attitudes toward fees. In the same vein, Biro and Hewson (1976) found that patients who made regular dental visits expressed more favorable attitudes toward care, more confidence in the dentist, and perceived greater interest on the dentist's part than did irregular users.

Ware et al. (1975) used a battery of multi-item scales to measure attitudes toward medical and dental services in seven southern Illinois counties. These measures, most of which pertained to medical care attitudes, were highly predictive of whether respondents (N = 903) made it a practice to see their dentist at least once a year. Respondents with favorable medical and dental attitudes reported this practice much more often.

Bene, Novasky, and Geldart (1974) reported that attitudes about access to care grew increasingly favorable as community size increased up to about 30,000 population; thereafter, somewhat fewer persons reported favorably about their access. Such a result may well reflect the tradeoffs between increasing availability of services as population grows and the perhaps longer waiting times for appointments or in the office in larger areas where more people are demanding services. Populations in larger areas may also differ from those in smaller areas in the standards they use to evaluate access experiences.

Scarrott (1969) noted that one-fifth of those who had changed dentists recently had done so because of dissatisfaction, although the primary reason for change was a household move. Similarly, Jenny et al. (1973) noted that 10 percent of the parents who were generally satisfied with their child's dental care indicated that they had considered changing dentists, largely because of some dissatisfaction with fees and/or office location.

SOCIODEMOGRAPHIC CORRELATES OF DENTAL SATISFACTION

Biro and Hewson (1976) and Fanning and Leppard (1973) both found that older people reported more favorable attitudes toward their dental care than did younger respondents; Biro and Hewson also noted that confidence in the dentist increased with age. Fanning and Leppard and Biro and Hewson both reported that women indicated greater fear of dental treatment than men. Scarrott (1969), studying aspects of dental care on which patients placed importance, noted few differences between social class groups or regions in Great Britain. Strauss (1976) noted several differences between blacks and whites receiving care in an urban dental school clinic in the United States, although significance tests were not reported. Blacks were more likely to avoid going to the dentist because they feared pain from treatment, more likely to respect the dentist, less likely to report having seen a cruel, rough or inconsiderate dentist, and less apt than whites to believe there were enough dentists available in the community. Similar proportions (about 25 percent) of both groups thought dental fees were "about right."

SUMMARY

Our literature review indicates that satisfaction with dental care has been viewed as a multidimensional concept. The dimensions revealed in content analyses of satisfaction measures and in empirical tests of dimensionality include: quality of care (both interpersonal and technical aspects), accessibility (financial and nonfinancial), availability, convenience, pain management, general satisfaction, practice organization, specific features of treatment, efficacy/outcomes, and continuity of provider.

Investigators infrequently reported variability for dental satisfaction measures. When descriptive statistics were available, means tended to be on the side of the score midpoint indicating favorable attitudes toward dental care and providers. Variability appeared to be adequate (again, when reported) for correlational analyses.

Information about reliablity of dental satisfaction measures, although sparse, indicates that multi-item measures are reliable enough for group comparisons. Without more information about reliability, it is difficult to place much weight on the magnitudes of the few validity coefficients that we found in the literature. Therefore, it is hard to determine how successful all published studies have been in actually measuring patient satisfaction. The evidence of content validity for most measures we found is favorable, and the little empirical evidence thus far available from cross-sectional studies generally supports the validity of the measures. However, the evidence is far short of what is needed to rule out plausible alternative interpretations of scores on these measures, including attitudes toward medical care, general life sentiments, and (in some instances) such methodological artifacts as response set.

If we can generalize from the performance of satisfaction measures in the medical care area (Ware, Davies-Avery, and Stewart, 1978), we would expect additional empirical studies to support the validity of dental satisfaction measures, particularly those in the access (financial and nonfinancial), availability, and interpersonal areas. We believe that considerable work (both observational and experimental) will be required to understand the meaning of interpersonal and technical quality ratings in relation to other assessments of dental care quality; the same is true for the measurement of satisfaction with these aspects of medical care.

In conclusion, the patient satisfaction concept appears on its face to be a useful one for research on dental care providers and services. Further knowledge of the psychometric properties of dental care satisfaction measures, particularly their interpretation, is required to justify confidence in this conclusion.

III. DEVELOPMENT OF THE HIE DENTAL SATISFACTION QUESTIONNAIRE

ITEM DEVELOPMENT

The major dimensions of dental care satisfaction that we identified in the literature include quality of care (both interpersonal and technical aspects), accessibility (financial and nonfinancial) and availability, convenience, and pain management. Less commonly measured dimensions were general satisfaction with dental care, practice organization, specific features of treatment, efficacy/outcomes, and continuity.

With the exception of pain management, practice organization, and features of treatment, the above-listed dimensions were also represented in a 43-item battery designed to measure patient satisfaction with medical care already being used in HIE health questionnaires (Ware, Snyder, and Wright, 1976). Given our knowledge of the psychometric properties of items in that battery, we adapted items from them for the DSQ by changing item references from medical care and physicians to dental care and dentists. We selected items for this adaptation from the scales in the medical satisfaction battery that had been shown to measure quality of care (interpersonal and technical), accessibility (financial and nonfinancial), availability, convenience, continuity, efficacy/outcomes, and general satisfaction. New pain management items were written by project staff and reviewed by a dentist and other consultants.

Abbreviated item content for the 19-item DSQ is presented in Table 2.[1] A reproduction of the battery and directions to respondents as they appear in HIE health questionnaires are provided in App. A. Eighteen of the items are worded as complete statements of opinion about some aspect of dental care or dentists; one item (no. 12) is worded more as a statement of fact. Each is accompanied by five response categories ranging from "strongly agree" to "strongly disagree." This choice of response category assumes that each item is roughly neutral in terms of the sentiment it represents and that differences in attitude are reflected in the degree to which respondents agree or disagree. The battery includes both favorably and unfavorably worded statements. The direction of wording for each item is indicated in Table 2, as is its content category. Items are numbered in Table 2 and throughout this report in the order in which they appear in the dental satisfaction battery.

ADMINISTRATION OF THE DSQ IN THE HEALTH INSURANCE EXPERIMENT

The DSQ was designed for self-administration by HIE enrollees aged 14 and older, and requires an average of about 5 minutes to complete. This battery first appeared on the annual

---

[1] A 14-item dental care satisfaction battery was fielded on the second annual Health Questionnaire (HQ #2) administered in Dayton at the end of that site's first year of experience with dental benefits. This preliminary battery was only fielded once, and was later expanded to the 19-item version to improve content validity. The 14-item battery was not analyzed separately and is not discussed in this report. We did develop scoring rules that allow the same major satisfaction dimensions to be scored from the 14- and 19-item batteries. These rules, which are reproduced in App. B along with the 14-item battery, will be used to score Dayton HQ #2 data on dental satisfaction for experimental analyses.

Table 2

ABBREVIATED ITEM CONTENT, DIRECTION OF WORDING, AND
CONTENT CATEGORY, DENTAL SATISFACTION ITEMS

Item	Abbreviated Content	Direction of Wording	Content Category
1	Dental care could be better	−	General
2	Dentists check everything	+	Technical
3	Fees too high	−	Financial
4	Avoid dentist because painful	−	Pain
5	Wait long time at dentist's office	−	Access
6	Dentists treat patients with respect	+	Interpersonal
7	Enough dentists around here	+	Availability
8	Dentists should reduce pain	−	Pain
9	Dental care conveniently located	+	Convenience
10	Dentists avoid unnecessary expenses	+	Financial
11	Dentists not thorough	−	Technical
12	See same dentist	+	Continuity
13	Hard to get appointment	−	Access
14	Dentists relieve most problems	+	Outcomes
15	Office hours good	+	Access
16	Dentists explain what they do and cost	+	Interpersonal
17	Keep people from problems with teeth	+	Prevention
18	Dentists' offices modern	+	Technical
19	Not concerned about pain	+	Pain

Health Questionnaire (HQ) fielded at the end of the first experimental year in Seattle, Massachusetts, and South Carolina. The DSQ appeared on alternate HQs in these three sites, on the fourth annual HQ fielded in Dayton, and on exit Medical History Questionnaires (MHQ) in all sites.

Placement of the battery within the questionnaires varied somewhat, depending on the length of the questionnaire. In addition, its placement was varied intentionally in the first HQ fielded in Seattle, Massachusetts, and South Carolina. A random half of the sample completed the battery before answering questions about health status, and the other half completed it at the end of their HQ. This randomized-groups experiment was done to examine the possible effects of questionnaire placement on both mean scores and response error.

IV. METHODS

DATA-GATHERING METHODS

Data reported in this volume came from responses to the first questionnaire fielded in each of the HIE sites that included the 19-item DSQ. In one site (Dayton, Ohio), this battery first appeared on the self-administered exit MHQ for the three-year sample.[1] In the other HIE sites, the 19-item battery appeared on the first annual HQ.

Because of its length, the self-administered MHQ was divided into two booklets (Form A and Form B). All adults completed Form A in their homes before the experimental intervention began and again on exit from the study. Those who did not receive the medical screening examination at enrollment also completed Form B of the MHQ at home (Smith et al., 1978). Adults who were screened at enrollment and all adults at exit completed Form B at the screening center in their site.[2] Health Questionnaires, which contained a subset of the MHQ health status batteries and were fielded annually near the anniversary of enrollment date, were also self-administered at home by enrollees aged 14 and older.

Each family head who completed the exit MHQ and screening exam received a $20.00 compensation, up to a maximum per family of $50.00. The family maximum included a $5.00 compensation for each MHQ completed for dependents (chiefly children aged 13 and under). Families received $5.00 per family head for completing the annual HQs.

Questionnaires were carefully checked for missing responses against stringent field-edit specifications. Respondents were contacted if responses were missing on more than six items (out of many hundreds), and the missing information was obtained over the telephone. If the respondent had problems answering the questions, interviewer assistance was provided. When the usually self-administered questionnaire was interviewer-administered, this difference was noted in the data base. Data were processed using standardized coding procedures and "cleaned" by a computer program that checked for possible coding errors and assigned a data status indicator that described data quality for each item in the questionnaire.

SAMPLE CHARACTERISTICS

Table 3 presents selected characteristics of the 3464 respondents (aged 14 and older) at each HIE site and across sites who provided data for dental care satisfaction measures on the MHQs and HQs described above.[3] As the table indicates, the analytic sample had slightly

---

[1]Approximately 70 percent of the sample is enrolled for three years and the remainder for five years. Differences in length of enrollment will permit analyses of the responsiveness of demand for services to enrollment period.

[2]Some HIE enrollees had moved out of the experimental site before their participation ended. These enrollees completed exit procedures in their new locations; questionnaires were usually completed at home and screening examination tests in their local doctors' offices.

[3]For these analyses, the Seattle sample excludes the control group that receives care from a prepaid group practice. The HIE randomly assigned some experimental families to receive care from a prepaid group practice in Seattle, and identified as a control group families that met eligibility criteria but had already chosen the group practice. Because of the possible self-selection bias (e.g., healthier families choosing the group practice), control group data were not used in scaling studies. The South Carolina sample includes the pre-experimental group (a sample intended for three-year enrollment) that self-administered the MHQ when the five-year South Carolina sample enrolled. In all sites but South Carolina, the three- and five-year samples enrolled at the same time and exited two years apart. In South Carolina, the five-year sample began participating two years before the three-year group, and the two will exit simultaneously. Because of these differences in sample definition, the sample sizes

Table 3

SUMMARY OF SAMPLE CHARACTERISTICS FOR ANALYSES
OF DENTAL SATISFACTION MEASURES

Characteristics	All Sites Combined	Dayton	Seattle	Massachusetts[a]	South Carolina[b]
Sample Size	3464	373	1654	1129	308
Age (years)					
Mean	32.8	35.8	32.5	33.6	30.4
Range	14-79	14-64	14-61	14-79	14-59
Sex (%)					
Male	47.4	45.6	48.4	47.1	45.2
Female	52.6	54.4	51.6	52.9	54.8
Race (%)[c]					
Nonwhite	8.1	13.6	4.8	1.8	44.5
White	91.9	86.5	95.2	98.3	55.5
Education (years)[d]					
Mean	12.5	12.6	12.8	12.4	11.3
Range	2-25	3-24	4-25	2-22	2-24
Family Income ($)[e]					
Mean	11,544	14,380	10,497	10,821	10,929
Range	0-55,893	0-55,893	0-35,000	0-28,866	400-29,917

[a]Combines Fitchburg and Franklin County samples.

[b]Combines Charleston and Georgetown County samples.

[c]Obtained for heads of household only.

[d]Obtained for respondents aged 18 and older only.

[e]1973 annual family income for Dayton; 1974 annual family income for Seattle, Massachusetts, and South Carolina.

more women than men, and was predominantly white; the South Carolina sample had the largest proportion of nonwhite enrollees (44.5 percent). Ages ranged from 14 to 79,[4] with a mean of 32.8 years in the combined-site sample; the Seattle sample was somewhat older and the South Carolina sample somewhat younger than the average. Education of family heads ranged from two to 25 years of schooling completed, with a combined sample mean of 12.5. Family incomes ranged from zero to $55,893, with a combined sample average of $11,544; families in Dayton reported the highest average annual income and those in Seattle, the lowest.

---

reported in Table 3 do not equal the enrollment sample sizes, and distributions of some characteristics may not exactly match those of the enrollment samples. Such differences are not likely to have affected the scaling decisions made or conclusions drawn in this report. Here and elsewhere, samples at the two Massachusetts and two South Carolina sites have been combined.

[4]A small number of persons older than 61 who were in eligible families were enrolled in the HIE but are not themselves eligible for insurance benefits. Although data are collected from these people and are used in scaling studies, they will not be included in the experimental analyses.

ANALYSIS PLAN

Studies of the HIE dental care satisfaction measures were designed to evaluate whether the battery would yield measures of the major satisfaction dimensions and an overall satisfaction index, and to determine whether the measures would yield variable, reliable, and valid scores. We also examined possible threats to validity from response sets, and the effects of questionnaire placement on score means and reliability. The methods we used to construct scales and to study validity and response sets are discussed in detail after the analysis plan. The analytic steps done to evaluate the battery are described below in order of their presentation in the results:

1. Examine item variability.
2. Evaluate the scaling and scoring of item groupings hypothesized to assess Access, Availability/Convenience, Cost (financial access), Pain Management, and Quality.
3. Evaluate a summary Access scale that aggregates the subdimensions of this construct (i.e., nonfinancial access, availability/convenience, and financial access).
4. Evaluate a summary index that reflects all the dimensions of dental satisfaction assessed by the subscales.
5. Report descriptive statistics for the dental satisfaction measures.
6. Estimate reliability for all measures in each HIE site and across sites.
7. Estimate the effect of early versus late placement of the DSQ in the HQ on mean scores and on reliability by comparing means and reliability coefficients. The later the items appear in the questionnaire, the greater the respondent fatigue in answering those items.
8. Evaluate the face and content validity of the dental care satisfaction measures in terms of their representativeness and comprehensiveness with respect to dimensions of satisfaction identified in the literature review.
9. Test the discriminant validity of the dental satisfaction measures by studying the relationships among the measures and studying their relationships with measures of other satisfaction constructs (i.e., satisfaction with medical care).
10. Address possible threats to validity from three types of response style: acquiescent response set, opposition response set, and socially desirable response set.
11. Examine the sociodemographic correlates of the measures.
12. Compare attitudes toward medical and dental care by examining differences in scores on medical and dental satisfaction items matched in terms of content.

METHODS OF ANALYSIS

Item Scoring

Before analyses began, each dental satisfaction item was scored so that a higher score indicated a more favorable attitude toward dental care. Missing responses were estimated whenever possible during the multitrait scaling analyses (see below). Scoring rules for all items appear in Table B.1.

Scale Construction Methods

Multitrait Scaling. Multitrait scaling,[5] a type of confirmatory item analysis, was used to test both the internal-consistency of the hypothesized scales that were defined in advance and the discriminant validity of items in those scales.[6] Respondents who did not answer at least one item in each hypothesized scale were excluded from multitrait analyses. Otherwise, scores for missing items were estimated for respondents included in these analyses by assigning each missing item the respondent's average score for other items in the same scale.[7]

We used two criteria to evaluate item-scale correlations, which had been corrected for overlap (using the technique recommended by Howard and Forehand, 1962). This correction provided more stringent tests of scaling criteria by removing the effect of the item being evaluated from the total scale score; because the scales we tested were short, each item had a considerable influence on the total scale.[8]

To satisfy the first (Likert-type or internal-consistency) criterion underlying the Method of Summated Ratings (Likert, 1932), uncorrected correlations between each item and its subscale should be substantial (at least 0.30) and positive. Similarly, to support scoring of an overall index, each item should also correlate substantially with the sum of all other items in the battery.

The second criterion, that of item discriminant validity, requires that the corrected correlation between an item and its hypothesized scale be higher than its correlations with other scales. In our analyses, the item discriminant validity criterion was satisfied and a scaling "success" counted each time the corrected correlation between an item and its own scale was more than two standard errors higher than its correlation with another scale. When the correlation between an item and another subscale was within two standard errors of its correlation with its own scale, a "probable" scaling error was counted. In such cases, we had reason to doubt whether correlations between items and their scales would be higher or lower than correlations with other scales upon replication. To take such marginal results into account, we defined and counted "probable" errors. Whenever the correlation between an item and its hypothesized scale was more than two standard errors below its correlation with another scale, we counted a "definite" scaling error.

Items that consistently account for definite scaling errors in discriminant validity tests are usually excluded from the scale in question. Inclusion or exclusion of items associated with probable scaling errors depends on several factors, including length of the battery, reliability of measurement, and the strength of associations between the constructs involved. An item that accounts for a probable error can be excluded, for example, if the battery includes enough other discriminating items to measure the construct that reliability is not adversely affected. If the intent is to construct separate measures of two constructs known to be substantially related (e.g., nonfinancial access and quality of care), probable errors associated

---

[5]This terminology has been used by Ware and others (1976, 1980) to refer to tests of item scalability that include multiple traits or constructs. This analytic strategy is not as complete as convergent-discriminant validation with the multitrait-multimethod matrix (Campbell and Fiske, 1959) because only one measurement method is represented. Multitrait scaling does extend beyond the traditional internal-consistency analyses because it provides discriminant tests of item validity across traits measured by the same method.

[6]We used a modified version of the Analysis of Item-Test Homogeneity (ANLITH) program developed by Thomas Gronek at IBM and Thomas Tyler at the Academic Computing Facility at Southern Illinois University.

[7]These procedures, which have been used in all HIE scaling studies, may have increased the internal consistency of the multi-item measures very slightly.

[8]For example, in the combined-site multitrait analysis, the uncorrected item-total correlations for items in the Access Scale were 0.79 (no. 13), 0.72 (no. 5), and 0.64 (no. 15). The corrected item-total correlations were, respectively, 0.41, 0.35, and 0.27. Because most studies report uncorrected item-total correlations, comparison between HIE results and those from other studies should note this difference.

with items in the two scale groupings may have to be tolerated at least early in the process of scale development and refinement.

Principal Components Analysis. After testing the hypothesized item groupings against multitrait criteria in a confirmatory analysis, we explored for unhypothesized dimensions in the dental satisfaction battery and evaluated the similarity of factor loadings for items in each grouping. We used the principal components method to extract factors from a matrix of correlations among the 19 dental satisfaction items with unities in the diagonal; all the variance in the items was considered in extracting factors. (Although use of item reliability estimates would have been preferable, they were not available when the factor analytic studies were done.) For the principal components analysis, items were *not* recoded. This has no effect on the absolute value of the factor loadings; the direction of loadings indicated the direction of item wording in the questionnaire, positive or negative.

The first unrotated component by definition accounts for the largest proportion of item variance and is therefore the most reliable one defined by the items. We evaluated this component for equality of loadings and to determine the dimensionality of the dental satisfaction battery. If only one important factor were identified (using the criterion that important factors have eigenvalues, or variances, of at least unity) and if all items measured the factor equally, homogeneity of measurement and simple scoring methods would be supported for all the items. If more than one important factor were extracted, or if correlations between equally reliable items and a given factor were unequal, more than one scale score would be required to adequately represent the constructs defined by the items (or some items should not be used to compute scale scores). The size of the first factor, in terms of variance accounted for, also gave us information about the appropriateness of scoring an overall Index.

Before rotation, we evaluated the initial (unrotated) principal components solution against several criteria[9] to determine how many factors should be retained and rotated to simple orthogonal structure, which makes interpretation of each factor more clear. These criteria indicated that from four to six factors should be considered in explaining the variance shared by the 19 DSQ items. We therefore compared conclusions across rotated solutions based on four, five, and six factors.

Reliability

We estimated the reliability of the multi-item scales with Cronbach's (1951) Alpha coefficient, which uses the internal-consistency approach. This approach treats common item variance as true score (reliable variance) and both unique item variance and random error as error. Calculation of Alpha uses data collected on a single administration of the items. At each level of item homogeneity (average inter-item correlation), scale length directly affects the magnitude of internal-consistency estimates. Therefore, we also computed homogeneity estimates for each scale to permit direct comparisons between scales that differed in the number of items.

Following Helmstadter's (1964) recommendations, we judged internal-consistency (Alpha) estimates of 0.50 or above to be appropriate for group comparisons. Such comparisons represent the primary use of dental satisfaction variables in testing HIE hypotheses about the effects of differences on coinsurance level.

---

[9]These criteria included the Scree Test (Cattell, 1966), the 5-percent guideline (Guertin and Bailey, 1970), identification of true common factors, and use of trial rotations. For discussion of these criteria, see Ware, Miller, and Snyder (1973) and Ware et al. (1980).

Because the internal-consistency approach is not appropriate for single-item measures, we used multiple correlations (communality estimates) to estimate the point-in-time reliability of the two single-item measures (General Satisfaction and Continuity). These estimates were obtained by regressing each of the single-item measures, separately, on all other dental satisfaction items. As Guertin and Bailey (1970, pp. 215-216) point out, the multiple correlation provides a lower-bound estimate of an item's reliability (because an item score may reflect unique reliable variance as well as common variance).

We calculated reliability estimates for each multi-item scale separately in each site and across sites. The sociodemographic characteristics of samples in the HIE sites differ, particularly on education and income, variables known to be related to data quality. Between-site comparisons of reliability estimates thus provided information relevant to whether reliability would be acceptable in the "worst case," when the poorest data quality might be expected.

Validity of Dental Satisfaction Measures

To understand the meaning of scores on the dental satisfaction measures, we relied on a construct validity approach, because there are no generally accepted criterion measures of these concepts. The construct validity approach involves examining patterns of relationships among measures of dental satisfaction and other variables to which they should (or should not) be related according to theory. More specifically, the construct validity approach requires empirical standards against which to evaluate the direction and magnitude of the observed relationships.

The literature provided little in the way of theory or empirical evidence about the relationships that would be expected for valid measures of the different dental care satisfaction constructs. We therefore began by examining patterns of relationships among the measures themselves, using a matrix of product-moment correlations among the DSQ scales, to test their discriminant validity. Our hypotheses at this stage of the analysis were that if the measures assess a common construct (i.e., general satisfaction with dental care) they should be significantly and positively interrelated. At the same time, if the scales assess distinct dimensions of dental satisfaction, as intended, these relationships should not be too strong; very substantial intercorrelations would indicate that the dimensions were not well distinguished by the different scales.

We also studied the extent to which these satisfaction measures distinguished dental from medical care. We hypothesized that to the extent the DSQ scales were valid measures of *dental* care experiences, they should correlate more highly among themselves than with measures designed to assess similar dimensions of medical care satisfaction. To test this hypothesis, we computed product-moment correlations among 10 item pairs, matched in terms of content (i.e., satisfaction construct) and differing only in their reference to dental or medical care services and providers, and did a principal components analysis of the items to examine their structure. We hypothesized two major factors corresponding to dental and medical care attitudes.

Methods of Studying Response Sets

We used the matched-pairs formula (Ware, 1978), which was based on Messick's formula (1961), to calculate acquiescent (ARS) and opposition (ORS) response set scores. This method requires pairs of items that are logically opposite (in terms of manifest content) and empirically opposite (substantially negatively correlated). Because the short length of the DSQ did not permit item pairs matched by construct and worded in opposite directions, we used such pairs of items fielded in the medical care satisfaction battery. Our approach required the assumption that if a given response style occurs for one attitudinal battery in a questionnaire, it tends to occur for another attitudinal battery. In the medical satisfaction battery, we identified four item pairs (see Table C.1) that were matched in terms of satisfaction construct and had high negative inter-item correlations.

Each instance of incompatible responses to items in one of these pairs represents an occurrence of acquiescence or opposition. For example, one matched pair contains two items that refer to availability of care: "enough doctors around here," and "big shortage of doctors around here." Respondents who selected affirmative responses ("strongly agree" or "agree") for both items manifested an acquiescent response pattern; those who selected negative responses ("disagree" or "strongly disagree") for both items manifested an opposition response pattern. Occasional inconsistent responses to items in these matched pairs could have occurred as a result of respondent errors in marking the questionnaire, random responding, or keypunch errors, and would not in themselves constitute evidence of response set. We were concerned about the consistent occurrence of such patterns across the matched pairs, and thus the potential confounding of DSQ scores with information about response set tendencies.

We counted the number of times ARS and ORS patterns occurred independently for each respondent; scores for each measure could range from zero (no set) to four (maximum set tendency). We next examined the consistency of the ARS and ORS response patterns for each respondent, and then correlated the set scores with respondent characteristics and with scores on the dental satisfaction measures. If the set scores were correlated with the satisfaction measures and with variables defining population subgroups, their effect would be to bias estimates of group differences. If the set scores were not correlated either with the measures or with group characteristics, further investigations of threats to validity from ARS and ORS would be unnecessary.

To estimate social desirability response set (SDRS), eight items adapted from the Comrey Personality Scales (Comrey, 1970) were interspersed in the mental health battery fielded on Medical History and Health Questionnaires. Table C.2 presents item wording and scoring details for the SDRS measure. Scores could range from zero (minimal SDRS tendency) to six (maximum SDRS tendency). Scoring studies of SDRS (Veit and Ware, forthcoming) indicate that this set occurs relatively consistently in HIE questionnaire responses. After computing SDRS scores for each respondent, we correlated SDRS with dental satisfaction scores and with variables defining group characteristics. We then examined the possible biasing effects of SDRS on group comparisons by separately regressing each dental satisfaction score on the sociodemographic variables with and without statistical control for SDRS.

V. RESULTS

This section presents results from analyses that were designed to evaluate the adequacy of the DSQ against the goals outlined in the Introduction. We report item descriptive statistics, examine the construction of multi-item scales from the 19-item battery, and present the results of reliability and validity studies. Our results also include comparisons of enrollee attitudes toward their dental and medical care services and providers, and the sociodemographic correlates of the DSQ measures. In Sec. VI, we discuss these results in relation to those reported for other dental satisfaction measures and their implications for use of the DSQ in HIE analyses.

DESCRIPTIVE STATISTICS: ITEMS

Before scoring and evaluating multi-item dental satisfaction measures, we examined descriptive statistics for the 19 items to be used in these scales. Our examination focused particularly on the comparability of item score distributions; roughly symmetrical (if not normal) response distributions with a mean of 3.00 and standard deviation near 1.00 (on a five-point response continuum) are desirable characteristics for items to be combined in summated ratings scales. In the results discussed below, all items had been scored so that a high score indicated a more favorable attitude; to accomplish this, the precoded responses were reversed for some items (see Table B.1 for details of item scoring procedures).

Means and standard deviations for the 19 DSQ items in the combined-sites sample appear in Table 4. Frequency distributions for item responses and descriptive statistics for each site can be found in Tables D.1 and D.2, respectively.

Response distributions for virtually all items were skewed, although we noted no tendency for respondents to select the most extreme response categories (see Table D.1). Means for 13 of the 19 items were on the side of the response scale midpoint (3.0) indicating more favorable ratings. The six items with means consistently at or below the midpoint across sites related to pain management (nos. 8 and 19), financial aspects of access (nos. 3 and 10), prevention (no. 17), and appointment availability (no. 13). The report of provider continuity (no. 12) had the highest mean across all sites.

Although standard deviations showed a considerable range across items, those for each item were very comparable across sites (see Table D.2). Moreover, standard deviations for 14 of the 19 the items were relatively close to 1.00. Those with the most restricted variability observed among these 19 items included the availability/convenience items (nos. 7 and 9), continuity (no. 12), efficacy/outcomes (no. 14), and respect (no. 6). Two of the pain items (nos. 4 and 19) had the most extreme variability observed for these items.

MISSING DATA

Respondents provided virtually complete data on all dental satisfaction items. From 90.9 to 97.6 percent of respondents in each site provided data that could be used in our scaling analyses. Most missing data occurred because the entire battery was missing (6.1 percent

Table 4

MEANS AND STANDARD DEVIATIONS, DENTAL SATISFACTION
ITEMS, ALL SITES COMBINED (N = 3252)

Item	Abbreviated Content	Mean	S.D.
1	Dental care could be better	3.24	1.02
2	Dentists check everything	3.63	0.81
3	Fees too high	2.29	0.92
4	Avoid dentist because painful	3.52	1.11
5	Wait long time at dentist's office	3.26	1.03
6	Dentists treat patients with respect	3.66	0.78
7	Enough dentists around here	3.52	0.80
8	Dentists should reduce pain	2.89	0.97
9	Dental care conveniently located	3.72	0.74
10	Dentists avoid unnecessary expenses	2.73	0.83
11	Dentists not thorough	3.41	0.84
12	See same dentist	4.03	0.86
13	Hard to get appointment	2.90	1.14
14	Dentists relieve most problems	3.85	0.64
15	Office hours good	3.43	0.93
16	Dentists explain what they do and cost	3.35	1.04
17	Keep people from problems with teeth	2.82	0.95
18	Dentists' offices modern	3.85	0.64
19	Not concerned about pain	2.64	1.21

NOTE: Items have been recoded so that higher scores indicate greater satisfaction.

overall; from 2.4 to 9.1 percent across sites). We cannot determine from information available at this time whether this level of nonresponse is related to complete form nonresponse or to nonresponse on the dental satisfaction battery. (Some battery nonresponse may have occurred by design; it was permissible on attitudinal batteries when the questionnaire was completed by a proxy respondent.)

When respondents completed any items in the battery, they completed virtually all items. Across all sites, only 0.001 percent of all possible responses were missing for those who completed any items. Because some respondents were excluded from analyses reported here because of missing data, the analytic samples were slightly smaller than those noted in Table 3. The combined-sites adult (aged 14 and older) sample numbered 3252; Dayton, 373; Seattle, 1654; Massachusetts, 1129; and South Carolina, 308.

SCALE CONSTRUCTION

Table 5 presents the multitrait correlation matrix from the cross-sites sample that we evaluated to test five multi-item subscales (Access, Availability/Convenience, Cost, Pain Management, and Quality); similar data for the two hypothesized aggregate scales (Access

Table 5

CORRELATIONS BETWEEN DSQ ITEMS AND HYPOTHESIZED SUBSCALES,
ALL SITES COMBINED (N = 3252)

Item Grouping/Item	Scale				
	ACC	AVCO	COST	PAIN	QUAL
Access					
13 Hard to get appointment	41*	23	29	18	29
5 Wait long time at dentist's office	35*	27	29	24	35
15 Office hours good	27*	22	23	15	30
Availability/Convenience					
7 Enough dentists around here	26	39*	13	15	28
9 Dental care conveniently located	30	39*	15	17	32
Cost					
3 Fees too high	32	12	40*	16	25
10 Dentists avoid unnecessary expenses	31	16	40*	14	33
Pain					
4 Avoid dentist because painful	22	16	14	51*	26
8 Dentists should reduce pain	26	22	19	48*	32
19 Not concerned about pain	13	08	10	39*	14
Quality					
2 Dentists check everything	28	25	26	16	56*
11 Dentists not thorough	33	26	29	23	54*
6 Dentists treat patients with respect	32	26	27	21	43*
18 Dentists' offices modern	19	23	07	16	36*
16 Dentists explain what they do and cost	25	16	21	14	34*
14 Dentists relieve most problems	20	20	08	10	30*
17 Keep people from problems with teeth	23	16	20	24	28*

NOTE: * indicates item-total correlation corrected for overlap; standard error of correlation equals 0.02.

Total and the overall Dental Satisfaction Index) appear in Table 6. Site-specific multitrait correlation matrices appear in Tables D.3-D.10. In these multitrait matrices, row entries represent correlations between each item and the sum of items in each hypothesized scale grouping. Asterisks indicate the hypothesized scale placement of each item and identify item-scale correlations that have been corrected for overlap as described by Howard and Forehand (1962). They represent correlations between an item and the sum of other items in its hypothesized scale. We did not include the general satisfaction (no. 1) or continuity (no. 12) items in the hypothesized multi-item scales. We did not expect the general satisfaction item to discriminate among the specific satisfaction constructs assessed by the DSQ, and considered the continuity item more a report of behavior than an attitudinal statement.

Analysis of Item Internal Consistency

Items in each of the five hypothesized subscales generally correlated at least 0.30 with the sum of other items in the scale, thus fulfilling the first (Likert-type) criterion of the

Table 6

CORRELATIONS BETWEEN DSQ ITEMS AND HYPOTHESIZED GLOBAL
SCALES, ALL SITES COMBINED (N = 3252)

		Scale			
	Item Grouping/Item	ACCTOT	PAIN	QUAL	DSI
Access Total					
13	Hard to get appointment	43*	18	29	41*
5	Wait long time at dentist's office	42*	24	35	46*
10	Dentists avoid unnecessary expenses	39*	14	34	39*
3	Fees too high	37*	17	25	36*
9	Dental care conveniently located	35*	17	32	39*
15	Office hours good	34*	15	31	35*
7	Enough dentists around here	31*	15	28	34*
Pain					
4	Avoid dentist because painful	25	51*	26	39*
8	Dentists should reduce pain	31	48*	32	45*
19	Not concerned about pain	15	39*	14	24*
Quality					
2	Dentists check everything	36	16	56*	50*
11	Dentists not thorough	40	23	54*	55*
6	Dentists treat patients with respect	39	21	43*	47*
18	Dentists' offices modern	22	16	36*	33*
16	Dentists explain what they do and cost	29	14	34*	34*
14	Dentists relieve most problems	22	10	30*	29*
17	Keep people from problems with teeth	28	24	28*	35*
Unhypothesized					
1	Dental care could be better	43	28	51	55*
12	See same dentist	28	16	28	34*

NOTE: * indicates item-total correlation corrected for overlap; standard error of the correlation equals 0.02; DSI = Dental Satisfaction Index.

multitrait analysis (see Table 5). The only exceptions to this criterion that we noted in the cross-sites analysis occurred for items 15 and 17 in the Access and Quality groupings, respectively. The site-specific analyses yielded similar findings; although the items involved were not always nos. 15 and 17, the items that failed to correlate at least 0.30 with their hypothesized scales were always Access and Quality items.

As data in Table 6 indicate, all hypothesized Access items correlated above 0.30 with the aggregate Access Total scale that we tested. Similar results were observed in site-specific analyses of this aggregate scale; only two items (nos. 7 and 15) failed to achieve the 0.30 criterion, one each in Massachusetts and South Carolina (see Tables D.9 and D.10). (We examined the hypothesized Quality and Pain scales again in Table 6 to provide scaling tests for Access Total and because these two scales represent the other "global" or aggregated constructs defined by the battery; this was particularly the case for Quality, which refers to both interpersonal and technical aspects of care.)

All items except nos. 14 (efficacy) and 19 (concern about pain) also correlated substantially with the sum of all 19 items in the battery, the hypothesized Dental Satisfaction Index (DSI) (see Table 6). These two items were among those with the most restricted variability observed, which may in part explain these low correlations. This finding also suggests that the two items may share less variance in common with others in the battery.

Analysis of Item Discriminant Validity

A summary of results from our evaluation of the discriminant validity criterion appears in Table 7. Recall that this criterion requires the correlation between an item and its hypothesized scale to be at least two standard errors (of the correlation) higher than correlations between the item and other scales. Entries in Table 7 indicate the number of times the criterion was met successfully; the total number of tests for each scale appears in the first column. The last row presents the number of successful tests across the scales in each site. In 68 tests of the discriminant validity criterion for the five subscales in the combined-sites sample, we counted 66 successes (97.1 percent).[1] These data indicate that the Availability/Convenience, Cost, Pain, and Quality items scaled perfectly in the combined-sites analysis. Across sites, success rates ranged from 69 to 98 percent. That these

Table 7

NUMBER OF ITEM DISCRIMINANT VALIDITY SUCCESSES FOR DENTAL SATISFACTION SCALES, BY SITE AND ALL SITES COMBINED

Measure	No. of Items	No. of Tests of Criterion	Successes by Site				
			Dayton	Seattle	Massachusetts	South Carolina	All Sites
Access	3	12	4	9	11	7	10
Availability/ Convenience	2	8	3	8	6	8	8
Cost	2	8	5	8	8	4	8
Pain	3	12	11	12	12	12	12
Quality	7	28	24	27	28	20	28
Access Total	7	14	9	10	11	8	12
Overall[a]		68	47	64	65	51	66

[a]Access Total successes are not included in the computation of the overall successes.

---

[1]Scaling successes and failures in relation to the discriminant validity criterion were defined in the Methods section.

errors were seen chiefly in the two smallest samples (Dayton and South Carolina) indicates that the errors reflect in part the greater imprecision of the estimated item-scale correlations in those samples. Although we focus on results from the combined-sites analysis here, we note major differences in the site-specific scaling results as we proceed.

In the combined-sites sample, two of the hypothesized Access items (nos. 5 and 15) correlated higher with Quality. Similar errors for these items were also observed in the site-by-site analyses. Most of the errors observed for the Access Total scale could thus be traced to discriminant validity problems for items in the Access subscale.

Although none of the hypothesized Quality items showed errors on the Access scale in the combined-sites analysis, several Quality items accounted for scaling errors on the Access scale in the site-specific analyses. From these analyses, it is difficult to determine whether to attribute the errors we observed to heterogeneity of the access and quality constructs, or to confounding of the two constructs in these items. The principal components analysis (see below) provided further information on this point. Although no other scaling errors were observed in the combined-sites analysis, several were seen in the site-specific analyses, particularly for items in the Access, Availability, and Cost groupings. Similar error patterns were obvious in our tests of the overall Access Total scale. Such errors suggest that the access construct has considerably greater heterogeneity than the others assessed by this battery.

The homogeneity (average inter-item) coefficients for the multi-item measures presented in Table 8 offer further evidence that the more global scales have greater heterogeneity. (Because these coefficients are not affected by scale length, they can be directly compared across scales.) As suggested earlier, the access construct is more heterogeneous than the others measured. In particular, aspects of nonfinancial access (cost) are less interrelated than are financial access or availability/convenience. This finding is consistent with the problems we noted earlier for the discriminant validity of items in the Access subscale. The heterogeneity of constructs aggregated in the overall DSI is also apparent from the low homogeneity coefficient for this scale.

Table 8

HOMOGENEITY ESTIMATES, DENTAL SATISFACTION SCALES, ALL SITES COMBINED

Scale	Homogeneity
Access	.27
Availability/Convenience	.39
Cost	.40
Access Total	.22
Pain Management	.37
Quality	.24
Dental Satisfaction Index	.19

Principal Components Analysis

To examine the multidimensional nature of the dental satisfaction concept and to explore for unhypothesized groupings among the 19 DSQ items, we did a principal components analysis on the matrix of inter-item correlations in the combined-sites sample. The first unrotated factor accounted for almost one-fourth of the common variance, and represented a bipolar general satisfaction dimension. All items, positively and negatively worded, correlated substantially (above 0.40, absolute value) with this first unrotated factor except item 19 (concern about pain). This finding again suggests that this item shares less common variance than others in the battery.

After evaluating the first unrotated factor, we rotated the statistically uncorrelated components so that their interpretation would be clearer. The Scree Test suggested that at least four important factors were defined by the 19 DSQ items. Five factors had eigenvalues greater than unity; six factors accounted for at least 5 percent of the total measured variance. Thus, depending on the criteria used to identify the appropriate number of components for rotation, from four to six factors are required to explain most of the variance shared by the 19 DSQ items. The cumulative amounts of variance explained in each item by one to six principal components are indicated in Table D.11, along with the percentages of total and common variance explained in all items by the different numbers of components. Across the items, from 42 to 66 percent of their variance was explained by the six common factors. Extraction and rotation of a second factor clearly would identify a distinct pain construct; the variance explained in the three pain items increased markedly with the second component. The rotation of a third factor would appear to increase the variance explained in items related to cost (financial access). On the basis of data in Table D.11, rotation of additional factors (beyond three) would not appear to be associated with marked increases in variance for items pertaining to any one satisfaction construct.[2]

On the basis of this evidence, we compared rotated solutions based on four, five, and six factors. None of these solutions identified dimensions of dental satisfaction that we had not hypothesized before the multitrait analyses. Rotation of more than four factors began to identify subdimensions of the quality grouping, which had the largest number of items. The sixth rotated factor was defined by only one item (continuity, no. 12). Because so few items were available to study these later factors, we focused on the four-factor solution, which of the solutions we compared provided the clearest information about the dimensionality of the DSQ items.

Correlations between the items and four rotated principal components are presented in Table 9. Items are listed in the table in order of their highest factor correlation, starting with Factor I. Correlations below 0.223 (absolute value), which accounted for less than 5 percent of an item's measured variance, were omitted to facilitate visual interpretation of the components and of item validity in relation to the four components. The right-hand column presents communality estimates, which indicate the proportion of variance explained in each item by these four factors.

The four factors generally represented the hypothesized quality, access (both financial and nonfinancial), availability/convenience, and pain constructs. The three hypothesized pain items defined a unique factor in all rotated solutions, supporting interpretation of a pain factor. The hypothesized quality items, as well as the general satisfaction item, correlated highest with the first rotated factor, supporting its interpretation as a quality factor. The one exception to the hypothesized quality dimension noted in the four-factor solution was item 17

---

[2]The second factor in the two-factor rotated solution *was* defined by the three pain items and the efficacy (no. 14) item; all other items had their primary loadings on the first factor. In the three-factor rotated solution, the factors were defined primarily by the quality, access, and pain items; we noted some overlap between the availability/convenience items and the quality factor in this solution.

Table 9

Correlations between DSQ Items and Four Rotated Principal Components, All Sites Combined

Item	Abbreviated Content[a]	Rotated Component				Communality
		I	II	III	IV	
2	Dentists check everything (Q)	79				66
11	Dentists not thorough (Q)	-74	22			62
1	Dental care could be better (G)	-59	31		23	50
6	Dentists treat patients with respect (Q)	48		28		36
18	Dentists' offices modern (Q)	48		37		42
14	Dentists relieve most problems (Q)	43		37		34
16	Dentists explain what they do and cost (Q)	42				23
17	Keep people from problems with teeth (Q)	32	27	32		28
3	Fees too high (C)	24	74			57
10	Dentists avoid unnecessary expenses (C)		66			50
13	Hard to get appointment (A)		55	-39		47
5	Wait long time at dentist's office (A)		43	34		38
9	Dental care conveniently located (AC)			68		48
7	Enough dentists around here (AC)			66		46
15	Office hours good (A)		-34	44		32
12	See same dentist (Cn)	28		42		27
4	Avoid dentist because painful (P)				77	63
8	Dentists should reduce pain (P)				75	63
19	Not concerned about pain (P)				69	46

[a] Abbreviation in parentheses indicates hypothesized scale placement for each item: Q=Quality; G=General Satisfaction; C=Cost; A=Access; AC=Availability/Convenience; Cn=Continuity; P=Pain.

(prevention), which had nearly equal correlations with the quality and pain factors. Rotation of additional factors indicated that this item primarily defined the quality dimension. Three of the quality items had noteworthy secondary correlations with the nonfinancial access or cost factor (Factor III).

The second and third factors appeared to be defined by access and availability/convenience items, respectively. The two cost (financial access) items correlated highest with the second factor, and the two availability/convenience items with the third. The nonfinancial access items were divided between these two factors; those with their highest correlation on one had substantial secondary correlations with the other.

Thus, the factor analytic results are consistent with the proposed multidimensional nature of the dental satisfaction construct. They provide strong support for the hypothesized pain and quality dimensions. The pattern of results also generally supports the hypothesized cost and availability/convenience dimensions, as well as an overall access dimension, but indicates the heterogeneity of the access construct. Overlap between the quality and access factors indicates, as did the item analysis, that there is some overlap between the access and quality constructs that are defined by these DSQ items. Supporting interpretation of the general satisfaction item as a general construct are its substantial correlations with the quality, access, and pain factors.

SCORING THE DSQ SCALES

On the basis of these results, we constructed seven multi-item scales. Five are multi-item subscales measuring financial (cost) and nonfinancial access, availability and convenience, pain management, and quality of care. A global access scale aggregates financial and nonfinancial aspects of access and availability. The DSI includes all items from the five subscales as well as the single-item measures of general satisfaction and continuity of dental care.

Three of the five subscales (Availability/Convenience, Pain, Quality) are completely consistent with both the factor analytic and multitrait scaling results. The factor analysis placed the cost and access items on the same factor. Most likely this is because these dimensions were not represented by enough items to permit derivation of separate factors. Our multitrait analyses, which are more appropriate for testing very short scales, supported the distinction between financial and nonfinancial (cost) aspects of access. This distinction is also supported by our content analysis and by the published literature.

To score all scales, items are first scored so that high item scores indicate more favorable attitudes toward dental care. Scores for relevant items are then simply summed to score the scale. Detailed scoring rules for all measures (items and scales) appear in Tables B.1 and B.2.

DESCRIPTIVE STATISTICS: DENTAL SATISFACTION SCALES

Descriptive statistics for the DSQ appear in Table 10. Site-specific data are presented in Table D.12. Frequency distributions for the scales in the combined sites sample follow in Tables D.13 to D.19. On all scales in all sites, observed mean scores tended to be higher than the midpoint of the possible score ranges, indicating that respondents scored on the favorable end of the scale. Despite the skewness observed, considerable variability was apparent in scores on all scales (data not presented here). The full range of possible scores was observed for all scales but Quality, on which all but the very lowest score was seen.

RELIABILITY OF SCALE SCORES

Reliability estimates for the DSQ measures in the combined-sites and site-specific samples appear in Table 11. For the multi-item scales, these estimates are internal-consistency (Alpha) coefficients (Cronbach, 1951); for the single-item measures, they are lower-bound estimates based on the multiple correlation coefficients from regressions of the item in question on all the other DSQ items.

Reliability coefficients for the multi-item DSQ scales and the General Satisfaction item ranged from 0.45 to 0.83 across all sites. Estimates for the more global Quality and Access Total scales were in the high 0.60s to middle 0.70s, and for the DSI, in the 0.80s across sites.

As expected, reliability was related to scale length and the observed homogeneity or heterogeneity of the dimensions. Longer scales (i.e., Quality, Access Total, and the DSI) were more reliable than the shorter scales. The reliability of the Access Total scale directly reflects its length, given the heterogeneity of the constructs within it.

The poor reliability of the single-item continuity measure reflects the fact that it shares

Table 10

MEANS, STANDARD DEVIATIONS, AND SCALE MIDPOINTS, DENTAL
SATISFACTION MEASURES, ALL SITES COMBINED

Measure	No. of Items	Scale Midpoint	Mean	S.D.
Access	3	9	9.60	2.24
Availability/Convenience	2	6	7.24	1.28
Cost	2	6	5.03	1.47
Access Total	7	21	21.86	3.72
Pain Management	2	6	9.05	2.52
Quality	7	21	24.57	3.40
Continuity	1	3	4.03	0.86
General Satisfaction	1	3	3.26	1.06
Dental Satisfaction Index	19	57	62.75	8.40

Table 11

RELIABILITY ESTIMATES[a] FOR DENTAL SATISFACTION SCALES,
ALL SITES COMBINED AND BY SITE

Measure	No. of Items	All Sites Combined	Site			
			Dayton	Seattle	Massachusetts	South Carolina
Access	3	.52	.45	.51	.57	.52
Availability/Convenience	2	.56	.50	.55	.52	.62
Cost	2	.57	.60	.57	.57	.53
Access Total	7	.66	.68	.66	.67	.65
Pain Management	2	.64	.61	.65	.67	.59
Quality	7	.68	.74	.68	.68	.66
Continuity	1	.38	(b)	(b)	(b)	(b)
General Satisfaction	1	.60	(b)	(b)	(b)	(b)
Dental Satisfaction Index	19	.81	.83	.81	.81	.80

[a] For multi-item scales, coefficients are internal-consistency (Alpha) reliability estimates; for single-item scales, estimates are square roots of estimated communalities (see Methods for more detail).

[b] Not available.

less common variance with the remaining items in the battery, as evidenced by its notably low loading on the first unrotated component. Because of this, the communality estimate represents a lower-bound estimate of true reliability. Although we expect its actual reliability to be higher than this estimate, it may well not achieve the 0.50 standard for group comparisons unless other items are added and a multi-item scale can be constructed. Single-item satisfaction measures are usually notably less reliable than well-constructed multi-item scales (Ware, Snyder, and Wright, 1976).

Samples in the HIE sites differ in several sociodemographic characteristics, particularly education and income, that are related to data quality. Reliability often is poorer in less advantaged samples. To examine reliability of the DSQ scales in the "worst" site, we compared reliability estimates across the sites (see site-specific columns in Table 11). With one exception, internal-consistency reliability coefficients for all multi-item scales were at or above 0.50 in each site studied. The single exception occurred for Access, one of the shorter and more heterogeneous scales, in Dayton. We observed no consistent (across measures) trends to indicate that the measures were less reliable in South Carolina, the site with the least advantaged sample. Median reliability estimates across all scales in each site were in the low 0.60s.

EFFECT OF QUESTIONNAIRE PLACEMENT

The effect of questionnaire placement on scale scores and measurement reliability was examined by varying the placement of the DSQ in a randomized-groups experiment. The DSQ was presented in the midst of some 300 health status items in half the sample's self-administered first annual HQ (Form I), and as the last battery for the other half (Form II). Mean scores for the DSQ measures in each form appear in Table 12 for Massachusetts and South Carolina,[3] along with t-tests for the significance of the mean difference in scale scores computed for the two forms. Negative signs on the t-tests indicate that Form II means were higher, and thus that ratings were *more* favorable when the dental satisfaction battery was placed later in the questionnaire. The general pattern of results suggests that later questionnaire placement has the effect of slightly increasing mean scores on most measures except the Pain scale. From these data, however, the direction of the effect of questionnaire placement on mean scores for Access and Availability/Convenience cannot be firmly concluded. The increase was statistically significant (at $p < 0.05$) in both sites only for the Quality scale; mean differences were more apt to be significant in South Carolina.

Reliability estimates for scale scores computed for the two battery placements appear in Table 13. Reliability tended to be somewhat poorer when the DSQ appeared last, although the estimates indicated that reliability remained sufficiently high (above 0.50) to warrant use of the scales in group comparisons.

VALIDITY OF SCALE SCORES

A high degree of confidence in the meaning of DSQ scores requires the synthesis of several different types of validity studies. In addition, threats to validity from different response styles must be eliminated (or controlled) so the interpretation of scores is as little biased as possible. Results from the validity studies that we have done thus far generally support the validity of DSQ items and scales, although further tests of validity are needed. Our results also support the multidimensional model of satisfaction underlying construction of the DSQ.

---

[3]Although this experiment was conducted on the Seattle sample's first HQ as well, the data were not analyzed for this comparison because the response choices for several items were misprinted.

Table 12

EFFECT OF QUESTIONNAIRE PLACEMENT ON MEAN DENTAL
SATISFACTION SCORES, TWO SITES

Scale	No. of Items	Massachusetts			South Carolina		
		I (N = 542)	II (N = 517)	t^a	I (N = 139)	II (N = 137)	t^a
Access	3	9.84 (2.34)[b]	9.75 (2.14)	0.65	9.19 (1.96)	10.09 (1.99)	-3.76**
Availability/ Convenience	2	7.37 (1.25)	7.47 (1.26)	0.28	6.41 (1.60)	6.68 (1.47)	-1.47
Cost	2	4.93 (1.47)	5.07 (1.44)	-1.57	5.06 (1.30)	5.38 (1.38)	-1.99**
Access Total	7	22.14 (3.82)	22.29 (3.52)	-0.66	20.67 (3.67)	22.14 (3.31)	-3.49**
Pain Management	3	9.10 (2.63)	9.04 (2.49)	0.38	8.82 (2.42)	8.67 (2.32)	0.53
Quality	7	24.31 (3.49)	24.77 (3.18)	-2.25*	23.57 (3.15)	24.50 (3.27)	-2.41*
Dental Satisfaction Index	19	62.81 (8.65)	63.56 (7.80)	-1.48	59.87 (7.63)	62.28 (8.04)	-2.55*

NOTE: In Form I of the first annual HQ in each site, the DSQ was placed near the middle; in Form II, it was the last battery.

[a] t-test value for H_0: $\mu_I - \mu_{II} = 0$.

[b] Standard deviations in parentheses.

* $p < 0.05$, two-tailed test.

** $p < 0.01$, two-tailed test.

Face and Content Validity

To test face validity, we examined the wording of the DSQ items and found that they appear to measure the constructs they were intended to measure (as defined in Table 5). These constructs include quality (both interpersonal and technical aspects and efficacy), accessibility of care, availability and convenience of services, cost of care, and management of pain associated with dental treatment. Thus, the HIE items have face validity.

To test content validity, we compared the comprehensiveness of the DSQ items' content with that revealed in the literature. All known aspects of dental satisfaction except specific features of treatment and organization of practice are represented among the items (although not each aspect is scored separately). Although the continuity construct is represented, the item appears to measure behavior rather than satisfaction with continuity. The one continuity item we noted in the literature review (used by Scarrott, 1969) was a satisfaction item. Moreover, interpersonal aspects of the quality of care are underrepresented in the DSQ relative to the frequency with which this dimension has been measured in other studies. With these caveats, the items are generally comprehensive with respect to the content of dental satisfaction as revealed in the literature.

Table 13

EFFECT OF QUESTIONNAIRE PLACEMENT ON DENTAL SATISFACTION SCORE
RELIABILITY,[a] MULTI-ITEM MEASURES, TWO SITES

Measure	Massachusetts		South Carolina	
	I	II	I	II
Access	.62	.52	.50	.52
Availability/Convenience	.50	.54	.76	.44
Cost	.59	.56	.45	.55
Access Total	.69	.64	.70	.57
Pain Management	.69	.63	.63	.56
Quality	.70	.66	.64	.67
Dental Satisfaction Index	.83	.79	.79	.80

NOTE: In Form I of the first annual HQ in these sites, the DSQ was placed near the middle; in Form II, it was the last battery.

[a] Reliability estimates are internal-consistency reliability (Alpha) coefficients (Cronbach, 1951).

Construct Validity

Our multitrait item analyses and the factor analysis provided empirical evidence of the DSQ's construct validity in relation to its hypothesized internal structure. Results of both types of analysis confirmed the groupings of items hypothesized to measure the same satisfaction dimension, and generally supported the discriminant validity of the items in relation to those dimensions. The factor analysis and analyses of item homogeneity also indicated the multidimensional nature of the dental satisfaction construct. We identified a general factor common to all DSQ items, supporting our decision to score the DSI. However, four to six factors, generally corresponding to the hypothesized DSQ subscales, were necessary to explain most of the variance in item scores. Moreover, the notably lower homogeneity of the DSI than its component subscales indicated that some clusters of items share more variance in common than others. Thus, a single-factor or unidimensional model does *not* fully explain the relationships among the items, despite the overlap we observed among items in the item analyses and factors in the factor analysis.

Analyses of correlations among the DSQ scales provide further evidence of the dimensionality of the dental satisfaction construct. Were the scales simply alternate-form measures of the same construct, we would expect their intercorrelations to approach their reliability estimates (the reliability of two alternate-form measures is estimated by their intercorrelation). As can be seen from Table 14, the DSQ scales measure different but related constructs. Correlations between the multi-item measures in the combined-sites sample range in magnitude from 0.15 to 0.43, with a median of 0.34; reliability estimates for these measures (which appear in the diagonal of Table 14) range from 0.52 to 0.68, with a median of 0.56. (Correla-

Table 14

Correlations among Dental Satisfaction Scales

Scale	ACSS	COST	AVCO	ACST	PAIN	QUAL	CONT	GSAT	DSI
Access (ACSS)	(.52)								
Cost (COST)	.37	(.57)							
Availability/ Convenience (AVCO)	.33	.15	(.56)						
Access Total (ACST)	.47*	.35*	.31*	(.66)					
Pain (PAIN)	.26	.18	.19	.29	(.64)				
Quality (QUAL)	.43	.34	.36	.52	.30	(.68)			
Continuity (CONT)	.25	.14	.21	.28	.16	.28	(.35)		
General Satisfaction (GSAT)	.34	.33	.26	.43	.28	.51	.24	(.60)	
Dental Satisfaction Index (DSI)	.52*	.40*	.40*	.56*	.36*	.58*	.33*	.55*	(.81)

NOTE: Reliability estimates appear in the diagonal; all correlations are significant at $p < 0.001$; N = 3624.

*Correlation adjusted for effects of relevant item inclusion (e.g., the three Access items are used in scoring Access Total: the ACSS-ACST correlation is that between the three-item Access scale and the sum of the remaining four items in Access Total).

tions marked with an asterisk '*' in Table 14 indicate those that have been adjusted for overlap.)

The correlations clearly indicate that financial aspects of access are distinct from aspects of availability and convenience ($r = 0.15$), providing discriminant evidence of validity for these two access-related measures. The other pair of access scales (Access and Availability/Convenience) were more closely related. As hypothesized during scaling studies, the General Satisfaction measure did not discriminate among the satisfaction constructs. Although it correlated highest with the Quality scale, it had generally substantial correlations with all the scales. This pattern of results supports its interpretation as a measure of overall, or general, satisfaction with dental care.

As we noted earlier, the wording of the Continuity item suggests that it assesses actual behavior rather than attitude toward seeing the same provider on every visit. Its correlations with the other DSQ measures suggest that this item, although related to satisfaction (particularly with access and quality), may be a distinct concept. Supporting this contention are its low correlations with most satisfaction measures (ranging from 0.14 to 0.28); it had an adjusted correlation of 0.33 with the Index, which suggests that continuity and overall satisfaction are related in the hypothesized direction. While its low intercorrelations with the other DSQ measures may be explained in part by the low reliability of the single-item Continuity measure, the factor analysis provided further evidence that this measure assessed a concept somewhat distinct from the others assessed by the DSQ battery. As noted earlier, the fifth factor was defined principally by this one item; all others had negligible correlations with this factor.

Similarly, the Pain Management scale is somewhat less related to the other satisfaction measures than they are among themselves. Its interscale correlations were generally low to moderate, ranging from 0.16 to 0.30, and 0.36 for the DSI. Further analysis of the meaning of this measure is necessary to determine whether pain management is a distinct aspect of satisfaction, or a related but theoretically distinct concept in its own right.

Regression analyses that took correlations among the scales into account offer further support for the discriminant validity of the scales, and for the multidimensional conceptualization of dental satisfaction. We regressed the General Satisfaction item on the other subscales (Access, Availability/Convenience, Cost, Continuity, Quality, and Pain Management). Unstandardized (UNS) and standardized (STD) regression coefficients for the measures appear in Table 15; the zero-order correlations appeared in Table 14. The unstandardized coefficients indicate the change in scale units for General Satisfaction scores that is associated with a one-unit scale score change on each of the satisfaction dimensions. Standardized coefficients can be compared (keeping in mind the different reliabilities of the measures) to identify the more important satisfaction dimensions.

The squared multiple correlation from this predictive equation was 0.32, indicating that the scales explain about one-third of the measured variance and just over half of the reliable variance in the single-item General Satisfaction rating. The t-statistic associated with the regression coefficient for each DSQ scale was significant in this regression (see Table 15). In other words, each scale makes a significant contribution to the prediction of General Satisfaction scores. Thus, each of the constructs assessed by the subscales has a unique relationship with the general dimension, apart from the variance it shares in common with the other satisfaction constructs. Comparison of the standardized coefficients suggests that quality, cost, and continuity are the most important predictors of general satisfaction.

Table 15

UNSTANDARDIZED AND STANDARDIZED REGRESSION COEFFICIENTS FOR PREDICTION OF GENERAL SATISFACTION WITH DENTAL CARE, BY DIMENSIONS OF DENTAL SATISFACTION

Measures of Dimensions	Coefficients		t^a
	UNSTD	STD	
Access	.07	.03	3.90
Availability/Convenience	.05	.04	3.00
Cost	.14	.10	8.56
Pain Management	.10	.04	6.12
Quality	.37	.11	20.78
Continuity	.08	.10	5.26

[a] t-statistic for each coefficient is significant at $p < 0.01$, one-tailed test.

As noted earlier, many DSQ items were constructed by adapting items that are used to measure patient satisfaction with medical care. This adaptation yielded 10 item pairs that differ only in their reference to type of care and provider, dental or medical. We examined correlations within and between the two sets of items to further test the validity of the DSQ measures. The full correlation matrix appears in Table 16; items were not recoded for this analysis, so correlations between items worded in different directions have negative signs. The upper left-hand and lower right-hand portions of the matrix provide correlations among the dental and medical satisfaction items, respectively; because these two parts of the matrix are symmetric, their upper halves are not reproduced. Correlations between pairs of dental and medical satisfaction items appear in the lower left-hand portion of the full matrix. To evaluate correlations between matched dental and medical items (underlined in the diagonal of the lower left-hand part of the matrix), the magnitude of their correlations with items in their own set (medical or dental) must also be considered. We expected the dental and the medical items, respectively, to be more highly related among themselves than they would be with each other. In other words, correlations in the upper left-hand and lower right-hand matrices of Table 16 should be higher than those in the lower left-hand matrix.

Correlations among the 10 dental items ranged from 0.15 to 0.59, with a median of 0.25; those among the medical items were somewhat lower, ranging from 0.09 to 0.48, but had roughly the same median intercorrelation, 0.23, as the dental items. Correlations between medical and dental satisfaction items were notably lower in magnitude, ranging from 0.04 to 0.53, with a median of 0.15. These results suggest that the DSQ distinguishes aspects of dental care from medical care.

Correlations between matched pairs ranged from 0.20 to 0.53, with a median of 0.27. All correlations between the matched items were significant, indicating that people tend to have similar attitudes toward the same aspect of their dental and medical care.

Given the significance of these matched-item correlations and the similarity in magnitude of the median matched-item correlation with median correlations within each set of satisfaction items, an alternate explanation of these findings is plausible. The dental satisfaction items may not adequately distinguish attitudes toward dental care from those the respondents have toward medical care (and vice versa). Because the amount of information in the full matrix is difficult to synthesize visually, we also did a principal components analysis of the correlations among the medical and dental care items to evaluate the results in light of the two alternative interpretations of the full matrix. We extracted and rotated (to simple orthogonal structure) the first two principal components from the matrix in Table 16. If the items clearly distinguish dental and medical care, as we argue above, we would expect that the dental items would have their highest correlations with one of the first two factors and the medical items with the other. If the alternative explanation were true and the types of care (dental and medical) are not distinguished clearly by the sets of items, we would expect that the first two factors would define two major dimensions of satisfaction, with both the dental and medical items related to that dimension correlating highly with the factor.

The results of this principal components analysis appear in Table 17. As can readily be seen, the first two rotated components almost completely distinguish the dental and medical satisfaction constructs, which supports our conclusion that the dental (and medical) satisfaction items possess discriminant validity. For dental items, convergent validity loadings (i.e., loadings on the dental factor) ranged from 0.32 to 0.71, with a median of 0.52; secondary loadings (those on the medical factor) were notably lower, ranging from 0.01 to 0.36, with a median of 0.14. The pattern of noteworthy secondary correlations (those equal to or greater than 0.223, which account for at least 5 percent of an item's variance) indicates that some

Table 16
CORRELATIONS BETWEEN DENTAL AND MEDICAL SATISFACTION ITEMS, ALL SITES COMBINED

Items		Dental Items										Medical Items									
		A	B	C	D	E	F	G	H	I	J	K	L	M	N	O	P	Q	R	S	T
Dental																					
A Keeps patients waiting	(−)																				
B Fees	(−)	.25																			
C Convenient places	(+)	−.24	−.10																		
D Hard to get appointments	(−)	.35	.26	−.18																	
E Office hours good	(+)	−.18	−.18	.22	−.22																
F See same provider	(+)	−.22	−.12	.20	−.18	.15															
G Checks everything	(+)	−.24	−.20	.22	−.17	.20	.22														
H Not thorough enough	(−)	.31	.24	−.23	.21	−.18	−.22	−.59													
I Treats patients with respect	(+)	−.24	−.16	.25	−.21	.24	.21	.37	−.34												
J Care could be better	(−)	.32	.30	−.23	.26	−.16	−.25	−.46	.47	−.29											
Medical																					
K Keeps patients waiting	(−)	.28	.20	−.11	.23	−.16	−.07	−.13	.17	−.13	.17										
L Fees too high	(−)	.16	.46	−.07	.16	.12	−.05	−.10	.14	−.10	.17	.26									
M Convenient places	(+)	−.17	−.10	.36	−.20	.20	.08	.16	−.17	.19	−.15	−.16	−.12								
N Hard to get appointments	(−)	.18	.16	−.14	.25	−.16	−.07	−.12	.16	−.12	.16	.34	.22	−.18							
O Office hours good	(+)	−.10	−.14	.14	−.16	.53	.07	.16	−.11	.19	−.14	−.23	−.15	.22	−.24						
P See same provider	(+)	−.07	−.04	.11	−.06	.07	.20	.09	−.08	.11	−.14	−.13	−.09	.13	−.17	.14					
Q Checks everything	(+)	−.06	−.15	.09	−.18	.18	.05	.24	−.19	.24	−.15	−.24	−.20	.18	−.22	.24	.13				
R Not thorough enough	(−)	.15	.18	−.11	.20	−.16	−.09	−.17	.21	−.15	.20	.27	.27	−.16	.27	−.21	−.14	−.48			
S Treats patients with respect	(+)	−.07	−.09	.14	−.13	.20	.07	.22	−.18	.39	−.13	−.21	−.15	.22	−.17	.27	.19	.47	−.30		
T Care could be better	(−)	.13	.15	−.12	.18	−.17	−.05	−.19	.18	−.19	.26	.28	.21	−.17	.28	−.25	−.18	−.44	.46	−.36	

NOTE: N ranged from 3232 to 3245 because of missing data; items were <u>not</u> recoded for these analyses.

Table 17

FIRST TWO ROTATED PRINCIPAL COMPONENTS FROM MATCHED
DENTAL AND MEDICAL CARE SATISFACTION ITEMS

Abbreviated Item Content	Rotated Components		h^{2a}
	I	II	
Medical			
Checks everything	71		51
Care could be better	-69		48
Not thorough enough	-68		46
Treats patients with respect	62		39
Office hours good	53		30
Hard to get appointments	-51		28
Keeps patients waiting	-51		29
Fees too high	-42		20
Convenient places	32	28	18
See same provider	30		10
Dental			
Not thorough enough		-71	52
Care could be better		-68	48
Checks everything		68	48
Keeps patients waiting		-60	36
Treats patients with respect	26	52	33
See same provider		51	26
Convenient places		48	25
Hard to get appointments	-26	-44	26
Fees too high	-25	-39	22
Office hours good	36	32	23

NOTE: Decimals and loadings < 0.223 (accounting for less than 5 percent of the item's variance) were omitted.

[a] h^2 is a communality estimate, the proportion of each item's variance that is explained by these two components.

aspects of satisfaction with dental care (mostly in the access area) are less well discriminated from satisfaction with medical care than others; similar results were not observed for the medical satisfaction items.

Threats to Validity: Response Sets

Threats to validity may arise if the measures are correlated with response sets, tendencies to respond in some particular way to questionnaire items. Such response sets are particularly problematic if they are also correlated with sociodemographic variables, because the intended group comparisons may be biased as a result (Ware, 1978). Acquiescent (ARS) and opposition (ORS) response sets are manifested by tendencies to agree or disagree, respectively, with statements regardless of their actual content. Unlike ARS and ORS, the social desirability response set (SDRS) *is* related to item content, representing a tendency to select responses that put one in a favorable light or are socially acceptable given the question asked.

The DSQ scales were not significantly correlated with our measures of acquiescent and opposition response sets, because most were constructed to balance positively and negatively worded items. Ware (1978) has demonstrated that balanced scales do not correlate with response sets that are unrelated to item content. Thus, ARS and ORS are unlikely to bias group comparisons on the HIE dental satisfaction measures, and we did no further analyses of their effects on interpretation of these measures.

All the DSQ scales except Cost and Availability/Convenience showed low but significant correlations with the measure of SDRS. Moreover, SDRS tendency was more common among older, less educated respondents and women (see Table 18). To test whether these correlations with SDRS would cause us to reach different conclusions when comparing subgroups in a typical analysis, we regressed each of the DSQ subscales on the sociodemographic variables, with and without statistical control for SDRS. For each DSQ scale, conclusions about the existence and direction of group differences in satisfaction were the same regardless of whether SDRS was statistically controlled. Control for SDRS did affect (slightly) estimates of the magnitude of group differences in dental care satisfaction.

Table 18

CORRELATIONS BETWEEN SOCIAL DESIRABILITY RESPONSE SET AND DENTAL SATISFACTION MEASURES AND SOCIODEMOGRAPHIC VARIABLES

Measure	Correlation with SDRS
Dental Satisfaction	
Access	.06*
Availability/Convenience	.02
Cost	.02
Access Total	.05*
Pain Management	.10**
Quality	.11**
Continuity	.05*
General Satisfaction	.05*
Dental Satisfaction Index	.10**
Sociodemographic Variables	
Age	.10**
Sex	.05*
Race	.02
Education	-.13**
Income	.02

* $p < 0.01$.
** $p < 0.001$.

DIFFERENCES BETWEEN DENTAL AND MEDICAL CARE SATISFACTION

A comparison of mean scores based on the 10 matched dental and medical care satisfaction items in the combined-sites sample appears in Table 19. For this comparison, all items were scored so that higher scores indicate more favorable ratings. These comparisons showed statistically significant differences favoring dental care quality, office waiting times, convenience of location and hours, and continuity. Overall satisfaction ratings also favored dental care. No significant differences between dental and medical care satisfaction were found for fees or waits for appointments. We observed similar results in each of the sites except on the

Table 19

COMPARISON BETWEEN RATINGS OF DENTAL AND MEDICAL CARE ON MATCHED QUESTIONNAIRE ITEMS

Abbreviated Item Content[a]	Rating[b] Dental	Rating[b] Medical	Mean Difference	t
Accessibility				
Keeps patients waiting	3.28 (1.03)	2.50 (1.04)	0.78	37.78**
Fees too high	2.29 (0.93)	2.31 (0.97)	-0.03	-1.58
Convenient places	3.71 (0.74)	3.46 (0.89)	0.25	16.32**
Hard to get appointments	2.91 (1.15)	2.90 (1.11)	-0.01	-0.43
Office hours good	3.41 (0.95)	3.22 (0.97)	0.19	12.57**
Continuity				
See same provider	4.04 (0.86)	3.70 (0.94)	0.34	17.79**
Quality				
Checks everything	3.62 (0.81)	2.83 (0.92)	0.79	44.38**
Not thorough enough	3.42 (0.85)	2.97 (1.01)	0.45	22.97**
Treats patients with respect	3.65 (0.79)	3.31 (0.95)	0.34	20.98**
General Satisfaction				
Care could be better	3.22 (10.2)	2.76 (0.91)	0.47	24.02**

[a] Items differ only in reference to dental or medical care/dentist or doctor.

[b] Mean score with standard deviation in parentheses; higher score indicates more favorable rating.

** $p < 0.001$, two-tailed test of significance of mean difference.

appointment item (see Tables D.20-D.23). Respondents were significantly less satisfied with the time required to get dental appointments in South Carolina, and significantly more satisfied in Dayton; these findings may well reflect differential availability of medical and dental services in these sites. In South Carolina, we also we found no difference between continuity of dental and medical providers.

SOCIODEMOGRAPHIC CORRELATES OF DENTAL SATISFACTION MEASURES

Correlations between the dental satisfaction measures and five sociodemographic variables (age, sex, race, education, and income) appear in Table 20. We observed group differences, usually significant ones, on all but the Cost scale. Older persons were more satisfied than younger ones with the quality of their care and pain management, as well as with their care overall; no other age-related differences were significant. On all measures but Cost, nonwhites were less satisfied than whites with their dental care. Those with more income and who had completed more years of schooling were generally more satisfied with all aspects of their care but Quality; the Quality measure revealed no income- or education-group differences. Among the access measures, group differences were more notable on Availability/Convenience than on Access; no group differences were observed for the Cost measure. Although older persons reported no greater continuity of care than younger persons, women, whites, and those with more education and higher incomes were all more likely to see the same dentist than men, nonwhites, and less socioeconomically disadvantaged respondents.

Table 20

SOCIODEMOGRAPHIC CORRELATES OF DENTAL SATISFACTION MEASURES, ALL SITES COMBINED

Sociodemographic Characteristics	ACSS	AVCO	COST	ACST	PAIN	QUAL	CONT	GSAT	DSI
Age	.03	.03	-.01	.03	.11	.06	.03	.05	.08
Sex (female)	.04	.04	.01	.04	-.03	.07	.09	.11	.06
Race (nonwhite)	-.04	-.13	-.01	-.07	-.07	-.07	-.06	-.10	-.10
Education	.03	.07	.02	.05	.11	.00	.11	.06	.08
Income	.04	.06	.03	.06	.08	.02	.10	.05	.07

NOTE: Sex scored 1 = male, 2 = female; race scored 1 = white, 2 = nonwhite; ACSS = Access; AVCO = Availability/Convenience; ACST = Access Total; QUAL = Quality; CONT = Continuity; GSAT = General Satisfaction; DSI = Dental Satisfaction Index. Correlations ≥ 0.04 are significant at $p < 0.05$; those ≥ 0.05, at $p < 0.01$; those ≥ 0.07, at $p < 0.001$.

VI. DISCUSSION

At the outset of this report, we identified five goals that guided the development of dental satisfaction measures that would be used in HIE experimental analyses. These included (1) a short but comprehensive battery of items, (2) multi-item measures of the major satisfaction dimensions, (3) variability in scores on the measures, (4) sufficient reliability for group comparisons, and (5) valid measures. The preceding results indicate that these goals were generally met, although further work remains to be done to validate the measures. In this section, we discuss the results as they pertain to each of these goals and in relation to the literature, and make recommendations for further research and use of the DSQ.

COMPREHENSIVENESS OF MEASUREMENT

Our literature review identified 10 categories of item content among previously published dental satisfaction measures: technical aspects of care; art or interpersonal aspects of care; accessibility/convenience; finances; pain management; general satisfaction; practice organization; treatment features; efficacy/outcomes of care; and continuity. Among the 19 items in the DSQ developed for the HIE, all of these categories but practice organization and specific features of treatment are represented. Given constraints on the length of the battery (because it was added to questionnaires already containing several hundred health-related items), we judged the battery to be relatively comprehensive with respect to the content of items fielded by other investigators.

In the DSQ, quality is defined as how good the care is, both in terms of technical and interpersonal aspects of the care process. Accessibility refers to the physical and financial process of arranging for and getting dental care, including appointment and office waiting times. Availability refers to whether the necessary providers and services exist in the area, and to the convenience of location and hours. Pain management refers chiefly to how well the dentist handles the pain associated with dental treatment.

The DSQ does not include an item assessing each one of the aspects within the categories identified in our content analysis. For example, the interpersonal care item in the DSQ refers to respect; other aspects of this construct noted in the literature referred to the dentist's perceived sympathy, friendliness, and reassurance. (Below, we make specific recommendations about a more comprehensive measure of the interpersonal aspects of dental care.)

Thus, although the DSQ is fairly comprehensive and should prove useful in most studies, certain modifications or additions may make it even more so. If unique characteristics of providers or services not assessed by the current items hold analytic interest, other items of similar type and structure could be added. The content of other dental satisfaction measures can provide useful items (see Table 1), as may content analysis of measures assessing patient satisfaction with medical care (available in Ware, Snyder, and Wright, 1976). If the HIE measures are revised, scaling decisions and reliability should be reevaluated.

DIMENSIONALITY OF PATIENT SATISFACTION

The content analyses of responses to open-ended questions about consumers' attitudes toward dental care and the results of previous empirical studies that we found in the literature both supported a multidimensional conceptualization of dental satisfaction. These results suggested that there are distinct features of dental care and providers that influence patients' attitudes toward care. Because the favorableness or unfavorableness of attitudes may differ from dimension to dimension, they also suggested that measures of each one should be scored and interpreted separately before relying on any indicator that summarizes scores across those dimensions. Construction of multi-item indicators of the major satisfaction dimensions was therefore a major goal in our studies of the DSQ.

Studying the Dimensions

Our scaling studies yielded five subscale scores based on multi-item measures to assess quality of care (both technical and interpersonal aspects of care), nonfinancial access, availability/convenience, cost of care, and pain management. In addition, we constructed a measure that aggregates the three access-related subscales (access, availability/convenience, and cost), and an overall index that includes the five subscales and two single-item measures, one of continuity and the other of satisfaction with dental care in general. Results of the item and factor analyses done on HIE data thus supported both the multidimensional conceptualization of dental satisfaction and the hypothesized item groupings that assess each dimension. Although we noted some overlap between the dimensions in the scaling studies (particularly quality and nonfinancial access), they were clearly distinct enough to permit separate scoring and analysis.

Our empirical findings regarding dimensions of dental care satisfaction are consistent with those reported by Murray and Wiese (1975) and by Koslowsky, Bailit, and Valluzzo (1974). We suspect that the positive and negative dimensions reported by Hengst and Roghmann (1978) represent the effect of acquiescent response bias. The data they analyzed came from a sample of low-income respondents. Data quality is known to be poorer in less educated and lower income groups. In addition, tendencies to acquiesce—agree with items regardless of their content—can be pronounced in such samples. Extensive research on measures of patient satisfaction with medical care (Ware, 1977; Ware, 1978; Snyder and Ware, 1974) indicated that answers to questionnaire items were markedly influenced by methodological factors, particularly whether items were favorably or unfavorably worded. Ware (1978) noted that these influences were so great, particularly in data from socioeconomically disadvantaged samples, that the results of factor analyses of correlations among satisfaction items were better explained by differences in item wording (favorable or unfavorable) than by differences in the characteristics of physicians and medical care services described by the items. Acquiescent response set, which Hengst and Roghmann apparently did not consider, would explain the "methodologic" dimensions they observed, one defined by all the favorably worded items and the other by the unfavorably worded items. Statistical control for ARS and reliance on balanced multi-item scales largely eliminated these methodological artifacts from the scaling studies reported by Ware (1978), Snyder and Ware (1974), and by Winkler, Kanouse, and Ware (forthcoming).

Our second goal for the DSQ measures—construction of multi-item scales that assess the major satisfaction constructs—was thus generally fulfilled. This statement requires certain qualifications, however. The literature on satisfaction with dental care reflects considerable interest in the dentist-patient relationship (Collett, 1969; Sword, 1969; Zeman, 1969; Clark and Morton, 1977; Weinstein et al., 1978; Bernstein, Kleinknecht, and Alexander, 1979). In light of this interest, separate scoring and interpretation of the technical and interpersonal aspects of dental care quality would be useful. As we noted above, interpersonal aspects of quality are underrepresented by DSQ items, and we could not construct a separate multi-item measure of this construct. Addition of more items that assess this aspect of dental care could make the battery more useful to those who are interested in studying the major dimensions of patients' attitudes toward quality of dental care. Additional items might be selected from the content analysis we presented in Table 1, or might be adapted from those we have fielded in studies of satisfaction with art of medical care (see App. E).

Currently, the DSQ contains only one efficacy/outcomes item (no. 14), and we noted problems related to its constrained variability in HIE samples. Future studies might be well-advised to make the wording of this item more extreme in order to achieve greater variability. If interest in patient assessments of dental care quality continues to increase, as has that in patient ratings of medical care quality, additional items that assess attitudes toward dental care efficacy and outcomes may be useful.

As we noted several times in presenting the results, the item referring to dental care continuity (no. 12) appears to be more a report of behavior than an assessment of provider continuity. This item should be reworded, and perhaps others added to yield a reliable multi-item scale, if satisfaction with continuity is an object of measurement in future studies.

Scoring the Dimensions

The scoring rules that we tested for the multi-item DSQ measures involve computing the simple algebraic sum of item responses (following recoding as explained in App. B). These scoring methods should be appropriate for most analytic purposes. In other measurement studies (Davies and Ware, 1981), we compared simple summated ratings scores like those we tested here with scores based on standardized items and on factor scores. The latter two approaches are often recommended when item variances differ (as did those of the DSQ items) and when the items do not correlate roughly equally with their respective factors (again, as was true for some DSQ items). Our analyses indicated that the greater complexity in scoring introduced by item standardization or factor scoring improved reliability very little above that achieved by simple summated ratings scales. Given that experience, we recommend the simplest scoring rules possible for the DSQ measures.

Two measures—general satisfaction and continuity—are scored from single items. Although separate scoring and interpretation of these items may be of interest in many analyses, their poor reliability may preclude such an analysis. Addition of other items that assess these constructs, and construction of multi-item scales may be required. Despite their poorer reliability than the multi-item scales, we decided to score the two single-item measures, following the advice that a weaker measure of an interesting construct is better than no measure at all (Veit and Ware, forthcoming).

There is a definite tradeoff involved in choosing to analyze individual items, multi-item subscales, and aggregate indexes that summarize across satisfaction dimensions (subscales). The tradeoff is between the complexity and potential statistical problems with a separate analysis of each unit of information versus the simplicity and statistical power of more global measures. With aggregation, there is also the potential for loss of information and even distortion of results. For this reason, we recommend analysis of subscales before reliance on summary measures. If conclusions are consistent across subscales (e.g., Access, Cost, Availability/Convenience), it is appropriate to rely on and report results for a summary measure (e.g., Access Total). For the more heterogeneous constructs (e.g., access to care), an item-by-item analysis may be desirable to ensure that results are consistent across items within a subscale.

SCORE VARIABILITY

Scores on the HIE dental satisfaction measures were skewed in all the samples we studied. With the exception of scores on the Cost scale, scale scores were notably above the midpoint of the possible score range. Despite this skewness, we considered the observed score variability to be adequate for the correlational analyses we planned.

The skewed score distributions we observed for the HIE measures were very similar to those we noted for the few studies that reported descriptive statistics for other dental satisfaction measures (Murray and Wiese, 1975; Koslowsky, Bailit, and Valluzzo, 1974). Such skewness has nearly always been noted in studies of medical satisfaction measures, and appears to be somewhat more of a problem with dental satisfaction measures, given the greater favorableness of attitudes toward dental than medical care (see more discussion on this comparison below).

Others have interpreted favorable skewed scores such as these as indicative of generally high levels of satisfaction. For two reasons, this interpretation may not be correct. First, all the scores do is rank respondents. Where in that rank order satisfaction ends and dissatisfaction begins we do not yet know. One way to determine this point would be to use the Method of Equal Appearing Intervals (Thurstone and Chave, 1929) to construct satisfaction scales (for example, as Hulka et al., 1970, and Zyzanski, Hulka, and Cassel, 1974, did to develop measures of satisfaction with medical care). Another approach to identifying the point at which satisfaction becomes dissatisfaction would be to relate satisfaction scores to a wide range of criterion variables for which we would hypothesize different patterns of relationships for satisfied and dissatisfied dental patients; such studies have not yet been done in the dental satisfaction area.

Second, considerable experience with items like those in the DSQ indicates that the proportions of respondents scoring above and below the midpoint can be changed simply by varying the item wording to be more or less favorable (Ware, 1977), while holding the satisfaction dimension constant. For example, one way to reduce the skewness of score distributions would be to make favorably worded items even more extreme; respondents would be more apt to choose somewhat less favorable response choices when indicating their attitudes.

The variability we observed suggests that the DSQ scales will prove useful in tests of HIE hypotheses. This suggestion remains to be confirmed by analyses of their precision—by determining how large differences between groups must be to be detected by DSQ scales. Studies of HIE health status measures, developed using methods similar to those used in DSQ scaling, indicate that they are precise enough for HIE hypothesis-testing (Rogers, Williams, and Brook, 1979). Our finding from the construct validity studies that the dental satisfaction items distinguished between other dental constructs and medical care satisfaction constructs provides one line of evidence that supports optimism about the precision of these measures. Evaluating precision is a high priority for research on both dental and medical care satisfaction measures. Thus far, our literature reviews have not identified any published precision estimates for dental (or medical) care satisfaction measures.

RELIABILITY

Internal-consistency reliability estimates for the two- to seven-item subscales ranged from 0.52 to 0.68 in the combined-sites analysis; only one estimate below 0.50 was noted (for one of the shortest scales) in the site-by-site analyses. Lower-bound estimates of reliability for the two single-item measures indicated that General Satisfaction was notably more reliable than Continuity; the latter had a reliability estimate below 0.50. We found no reliability estimates for construct-specific dental satisfaction measures in the literature, so we cannot compare HIE results with earlier findings. These reliability coefficients are equal to or slightly lower than those estimated for measures of similar dimensions of medical care satisfaction (see Ware, Davies-Avery, and Stewart, 1978).

In all analyses, reliability estimates for the 19-item DSI were at or above 0.80. These estimates for the overall measure are very similar in magnitude to those reported for overall scales constructed by Murray and Wiese (1975) and Hengst and Roghmann (1978), which were also based on the summated ratings method.

Whether the estimated reliabilities are sufficient depends on the intended use of the scale scores. For the group comparisons planned for HIE analyses (or, for example, comparison of dental practices), a good minimum reliability standard is 0.50; for comparisons between individual patients, 0.90. Even the very short multi-item scales achieved or bettered the standard for group comparisons in all sites. Thus, to study group differences, which is by far the most common use of satisfaction measures, the multi-item DSQ measures and the single-item General Satisfaction scale are sufficiently reliable. As we noted above, our estimates of reliability for the continuity measure does not meet this standard in HIE samples. To the extent that this item contains unique reliable variance (i.e., variance not shared with other DSQ items), our estimate is biased downward. This possibility should be studied further before conclusions are drawn.

Although calculation of reliability estimates is a good idea (and a simple process) if the DSQ is fielded in other research, we expect that HIE results will be replicated in other studies using similar methods to field the DSQ. This conclusion is based on the consistency of our results across HIE sites.

Our analyses indicated that reliability estimates declined slightly when the DSQ was placed at the end of a fairly lengthy survey instrument rather than near the middle. Even more crucial to studies that compare groups, mean scores tended to be higher when DSQ items were administered near the end of HIE self-administered questionnaires. When analyzing DSQ scores, the placement of the battery must therefore be kept in mind. If its placement varies for respondent subgroups, comparisons between groups may be invalidated. If the order of administering the DSQ changes on different administrations over time for the same group, comparisons across time may also be invalidated.

Comparing reliability estimates across HIE sites that differ in sociodemographic characteristics, we found that reliability was not lower among less advantaged respondents. Our site-level analyses did not consider the "most" disadvantaged subsample in the HIE, which would have been the group with the lowest income or educational level. Because poorer data quality is a common finding for such respondents, however, we recommend that reliability be estimated separately for the "worst case" in future studies that use these measures, to determine whether group differences in score reliability seriously affect the precision of between-group comparisons.

VALIDITY

Our analyses of face and content validity yielded favorable results, indicating that the content of DSQ items is logically related to the constructs we intended them to assess, and represents virtually all the major categories of satisfaction identified in the literature. Item analyses and the factor analysis that we did during scaling studies provided discriminant evidence of item validity, suggesting that most items were more related to others in the same category than to those in other categories.

As we had expected, the general satisfaction item usually failed this discriminant test of validity; although its highest correlations were with the quality item grouping, it showed considerable overlap with the item groupings defining access and pain management. These results support its interpretation as a "general" satisfaction measure.

Further tests of construct validity came from analyses of scale intercorrelations and regression analyses using the separate measures to predict general satisfaction. These results generally suggested that although the measures are moderately intercorrelated, as might be expected if they measured the same concept, they distinguish different aspects of that concept, each of which makes a unique contribution to an overall dental satisfaction score.

The construct validity analyses, as well as the item scaling and factor analyses, called into question whether the pain construct defines one aspect of an overall satisfaction construct, or defines a unique but related construct. In the factor analyses, the pain items defined a distinct component of variance and had negligible secondary loadings on other factors. Taking reliability into account, correlations between the Pain scale and the other DSQ measures tended to be lower than those among the other DSQ measures. Moreover, although the Pain measure did make a unique contribution to predictions of General Satisfaction scores, its contribution was notably less than that of other (even less reliable) dental satisfaction constructs. This evidence begins to suggest that the pain measure may define a construct unique from but related to satisfaction with dental care, although it is by no means conclusive. Given the apparent importance of this construct to dental services research (see, for example, Fanning, 1973), its appropriate interpretation deserves more extensive evaluation than has been possible in the construct validity studies we have done thus far.

Another study of construct validity for dental satisfaction measures relied on external criteria; namely, matched items that assessed satisfaction with the same aspects of medical care. We first noted that the dental items correlated notably higher among themselves on average than with items that assess medical care satisfaction. Our principal components analysis of correlations among the matched and unmatched dental and medical satisfaction items identified two factors, one defined primarily by dental items and the other by medical items. Taken together, these findings indicated that the dental items distinguished the different features of dental care they were intended to assess, and moreover that attitudes toward given features of dental care are distinguished from those toward the same features of medical care.

We did note that certain dental items overlapped more with the medical satisfaction factor than did their medical counterparts with the dental factor; most referred to access-related aspects of dental care. The one medical satisfaction item that had a noteworthy secondary correlation on the dental factor also related to access. Such overlap is not inconsistent with our conclusion that the dental (and medical) satisfaction items possess discriminant validity, with respect both to different dimensions of care and to the two types of care. It is not unreasonable to assume, for example, that physicians and dentists organize to provide services in similar fashion and use similar considerations in setting fee schedules within given geographic areas. If this were the case, we would expect notable correlations between respondents' evaluations of dental and medical office waiting times and fees, as we observed in our results.

Another explanation may fit these findings; namely, that individuals have certain preferences for the organization and practice of their health care, and that the rating items measure these preferences rather than how care is organized and practiced. Were this explanation true, it would have serious implications for the interpretation of the DSQ scales as measures of attitudes about care, rather than preferences for care. The available evidence on this point pertains specifically to medical care satisfaction measures and suggests that preferences explain only a small part of the variance in these measures; the majority is explained by actual experiences with care (Ware, Snyder, and Wright, 1976).

Further evaluation of these different explanations will be possible with the HIE data base. For example, data on practice organization are collected annually from physicians and dentists in each study site. Data from the two provider types can be compared, and correlations computed between these objective measures and subjective evaluations of accessibility. Such analyses could provide more definitive information about the validity of the items in relation to known characteristics of the two types of care, and about similarities and differences in medical and dental care as a function of area.

We found no threats to the validity of HIE dental satisfaction measures from acquiescent or opposition response sets. A major assumption underlying our analysis was that if acquiescent or opposition response sets were manifested in one attitudinal battery contained in the HIE questionnaires (namely, the Medical Care Satisfaction battery), they would also affect the DSQ; we had no independent estimate of ARS or ORS for the DSQ. This assumption is not without precedent, although the literature on the subject does distinguish between response sets that affect given batteries and response styles that are manifest across batteries within a questionnaire. Because the effects of such methodological problems on dental satisfaction scores had not been reported in the literature published before our studies of the DSQ, further analyses of this issue with different dental satisfaction measures and battery-specific estimates of ARS and ORS would add to the confidence we have in this conclusion.

Although SDRS was correlated both with the HIE dental satisfaction measures (except Cost and Availability/Convenience) and sociodemographic characteristics of respondents (except race), the presence of SDRS did not change conclusions about the existence and direction of group differences on the satisfaction measures in a typical analysis. The bias slightly affected estimates of the size of group differences in dental satisfaction. Given these findings, and the considerable importance of precise estimates of such group differences in a policy study such as the HIE, we recommend statistical control for SDRS effects in analyses of group differences. As we indicated above, further study of the effects of response sets on dental satisfaction scores would be useful.

With the exception of studying the discriminant validity of dental satisfaction measures in relation to those of medical care, the validity analyses that we reported in this volume were all based on internal criteria, features of the relationships between and among items and scales. The evidence from these analyses is consistent with the validity of the DSQ scores, but does not prove they are valid measures of patient satisfaction with dental care. Two further lines of evidence must be evaluated, both of which depend on external criteria.

First, we need to know whether DSQ scores reflect known differences in the structure and process of dental care. Analyses of this issue would provide information about the validity of the dental satisfaction measures as dependent variables. The dental satisfaction literature that we reviewed contains little evidence relevant to this validity issue.

Second, we must investigate whether scores predict such behavior as use or nonuse of dental care services, which would provide information about their validity as independent variables. Most of the validity information we found in the literature was relevant to this issue, although the analyses of relationships between satisfaction and use were based on cross-sectional data, which are likely to yield biased estimates and leave unanswered the important question of causality. The best evidence relevant to this validity issue will come from longitudinal analyses, such as those that will be possible with data from the Health Insurance Experiment. Studies of both these validity issues are extremely important to the state of the art of measuring patient satisfaction with dental care.

COMPARING DENTAL AND MEDICAL CARE SATISFACTION

If the dental satisfaction measures are valid, the results of comparisons between matched dental and medical satisfaction items suggest that patients may be more satisfied with several aspects of their dental than medical care. Differences favoring dental care were particularly notable for items related to whether the provider checks everything and to office waiting times.

Although we have not examined empirically the possible explanations for these differences in favor of dental care, several come to mind. Data from studies on patient satisfaction with medical care indicate that respondents who have made more physician visits during the past year are often less satisfied with aspects of care related to accessibility and convenience (Ware, Davies-Avery, and Stewart, 1978). Because they encounter the system more often, they may experience an accumulation of problems related to arranging for and getting to care, and these experiences are reflected in their satisfaction scores. Data from the National Health Interview Surveys fielded in 1976, 1977, and 1978 (U.S. Department of Health, Education, and Welfare, 1979) indicate that persons visit physicians an average of about 4.8 times annually, while they make only 1.6 visits annually to dentists. Thus, differences in rates of utilization and amount of experience with access and convenience problems may explain some of the differences observed in medical and dental care satisfaction.

Dentists may also do a better job than physicians of organizing and scheduling their services to avoid unplanned delays and other access problems, although this does not appear to be the case in all study sites. Comparison of results across sites suggests that there are differences between areas of the country in the stress on dental and medical appointment systems. Although we noted no differences between ratings of dental and medical office waiting times in the cross-sites comparisons in Seattle and Massachusetts, we did find differences —in opposite directions—in Dayton and South Carolina. Respondents in Dayton evaluated dental office waiting times far more favorably than those for physician visits, while those in South Carolina rated physician office waits more favorably than those for dental care.

Real differences in the process and outcomes of the two types of care may also account for differences observed, particularly on the quality dimensions. We are beginning to accumulate evidence suggesting that patients can accurately report the medical procedures that occur during an office visit, and that the performance of medically appropriate procedures is related to patient evaluations of technical quality (Ware, Kane, Davies, and Brook, forthcoming). Some data relevant to this issue have also been reported in the dental literature (Lengkeek et al., 1979). Such information is consistent with the validity of patient evaluations of quality of care, although the issue needs far more study using both observational and experimental techniques to examine the relationship between what happens during care, patients' experiences of those events, and their evaluations of the care.

Another explanation for these findings may be differences in continuity of dental and medical care. The HIE data suggest that people are more apt to see the same dentist than the same physician for their care. Both longitudinal (Breslau and Reeb, 1975; Marquis, Davies, and Ware, forthcoming; Shortell, 1976; Becker et al., 1974) and cross-sectional studies (Kasteller et al., 1976; Shortell et al., 1977; Ware et al., 1975, 1976) indicate that individuals who see the same physician for the majority of their medical care are more satisfied with their care generally. We would hypothesize the same relationship between continuity of dental care provider and satisfaction. Thus, if provider continuity is greater in dental than medical care, we would expect attitudes toward dental care to be more favorable as a consequence.

GROUP DIFFERENCES IN DENTAL SATISFACTION

Our analyses of the sociodemographic correlates of the dental satisfaction measures indicate notable differences between age, education, income, and racial groups and between men and women on virtually all dimensions but the costs of dental care. This latter finding probably reflects the intended balance in sociodemographic characteristics across the experimental treatment plans, which would make cost (i.e., different coinsurance rates for dental care) uncorrelated with sociodemographic characteristics.

The group differences we observed generally indicated that older persons, women, more educated and higher income respondents, and whites evaluated most aspects of their dental care more favorably. These findings were comparable to those reported in the literature, particularly for the general satisfaction item and the overall index, since such measures were most often correlated with sociodemographic variables in other research (Fanning and Leppard, 1973; Biro and Hewson, 1976).

CONCLUSIONS

Our studies of the DSQ's measurement properties and findings reported thus far suggest that it fulfills the standards against which we evaluated its adequacy, and support its use in the HIE's experimental analyses. We have developed separate measures of the major dimensions of dental satisfaction, which yield good response variability and reliable scores. Variability is adequate for the intended correlational analyses and comparisons of group means, although the skewness of score distributions might be improved by item revision. The data on validity—the meaning of scores on the measures—offer initial support for their interpretation as indicators of the different dimensions of satisfaction that they were intended to assess. Of all the psychometric properties of the DSQ measures that we studied, the area with the most work remaining to be done is that of measurement validation. In particular, the validity of the measures as indicators of differences in structure and process of dental care and as predictors of dental health-related behavior requires considerable study, as does the status of the pain construct in relation to dental satisfaction.

We believe these results also support use of the DSQ in general population studies that focus on patients' viewpoints regarding dental care. Preliminary analyses suggested that patients may be more satisfied with most aspects of their dental care than medical care. Further research is required to better understand the meaning of these differences with respect to practice organization, process of care, and dental health-related behavior.

Appendix A

DENTAL SATISFACTION QUESTIONNAIRE

DENTAL CARE   19-item Battery

HERE ARE SOME THINGS PEOPLE SOMETIMES SAY ABOUT DENTISTS AND DENTAL CARE.

PLEASE READ EACH ONE CAREFULLY, KEEPING IN MIND THE DENTAL CARE YOU ARE RECEIVING NOW. IF YOU HAVE NOT RECEIVED DENTAL CARE RECENTLY, THINK ABOUT WHAT YOU WOULD *EXPECT* IF YOU NEEDED CARE TODAY.

PLEASE CIRCLE ONE OF THE NUMBERS ON EACH LINE TO INDICATE WHETHER YOU *STRONGLY AGREE* WITH THE STATEMENT, *AGREE* WITH IT, ARE *NOT SURE*, *DISAGREE*, OR *STRONGLY DISGREE*.

THERE ARE NO RIGHT OR WRONG ANSWERS. **WE JUST WANT YOUR OPINION.**

		Strongly Agree	Agree	Not Sure	Disagree	Strongly Disagree
1	There are things about the dental care I receive that could be better	1	2	3	4	5
2	Dentists are very careful to check everything when examining their patients	1	2	3	4	5
3	The fees dentists charge are too high	1	2	3	4	5
4	Sometimes I avoid going to the dentist because it is so painful	1	2	3	4	5
5	People are usually kept waiting a long time when they are at the dentist's office	1	2	3	4	5
6	Dentists always treat their patients with respect	1	2	3	4	5
7	There are enough dentists around here	1	2	3	4	5
8	Dentists should do more to reduce pain	1	2	3	4	5
9	Places where you can get dental care are very conveniently located	1	2	3	4	5

	Strongly Agree	Agree	Not Sure	Disagree	Strongly Disagree	
10 Dentists always avoid unnecessary patient expenses	1	2	3	4	5	13/
11 Dentists aren't as thorough as they should be	1	2	3	4	5	14/
12 I see the same dentist just about every time I go for dental care	1	2	3	4	5	15/
13 It's hard to get an appointment for dental care right away	1	2	3	4	5	16/
14 Dentists are able to relieve or cure most dental problems that people have	1	2	3	4	5	17/
15 Office hours when you can get dental care are good for most people	1	2	3	4	5	18/
16 Dentists usually explain what they are going to do and how much it will cost before they begin treatment	1	2	3	4	5	19/
17 Dentists should do more to keep people from having problems with their teeth	1	2	3	4	5	20/
18 Dentists' offices are very modern and up to date	1	2	3	4	5	21/
19 I am not concerned about feeling pain when I go for dental care	1	2	3	4	5	22/

CARD 06

DENTAL CARE 　　　14-item Battery

HERE ARE SOME THINGS PEOPLE SOMETIMES SAY ABOUT DENTISTS AND DENTAL CARE.

PLEASE READ EACH ONE CAREFULLY, KEEPING IN MIND THE DENTAL CARE YOU ARE RECEIVING NOW. IF YOU HAVE NOT RECEIVED DENTAL CARE RECENTLY, THINK ABOUT WHAT YOU WOULD *EXPECT* IF YOU NEEDED CARE TODAY.

PLEASE CIRCLE ONE OF THE NUMBERS ON EACH LINE TO INDICATE WHETHER YOU *STRONGLY AGREE* WITH THE STATEMENT, *AGREE* WITH IT, ARE *NOT SURE*, *DISAGREE*, OR *STRONGLY DISAGREE*.

THERE ARE NO RIGHT OR WRONG ANSWERS. **WE JUST WANT YOUR OPINION.**

		Strongly Agree	Agree	Not Sure	Disagree	Strongly Disagree
1.	There are things about the dental care I receive that could be better	1	2	3	4	5
2.	Dentists are very careful to check everything when examining their patients	1	2	3	4	5
3.	The fees dentists charge are too high	1	2	3	4	5
4.	Dentists always do their best to keep the patient from worrying	1	2	3	4	5
5.	People are usually kept waiting a long time when they are at the dentist's office	1	2	3	4	5
6.	Dentists always treat their patients with respect	1	2	3	4	5
7.	There are enough dentists around here	1	2	3	4	5
8.	Dentists should do more to keep from causing pain	1	2	3	4	5
9.	Places where you can get dental care are very conveniently located	1	2	3	4	5

		Strongly Agree	Agree	Not Sure	Disagree	Strongly Disagree	
10.	Dentists always avoid unnecessary patient expenses	1	2	3	4	5	22/
11.	Dentists aren't as thorough as they should be	1	2	3	4	5	23/
12.	I see the same dentist just about every time I go for dental care	1	2	3	4	5	24/
13.	In an emergency, it's very hard to get dental care quickly	1	2	3	4	5	25/
14.	Dentists are able to relieve or cure most dental problems that people have	1	2	3	4	5	26/

CARD 03

Appendix B

DSQ ITEM AND SCALE SCORING RULES

Table B.1

SCORING RULES FOR ITEMS,
19-ITEM DENTAL SATISFACTION QUESTIONNAIRE

Scoring	Item No.
1 = Strongly agree 2 = Agree 3 = Not sure 4 = Disagree 5 = Strongly disagree	1, 3, 4, 5, 8, 11, 13, 17
5 = Strongly agree 4 = Agree 3 = Not sure 2 = Disagree 1 = Strongly disagree	2, 6, 7, 9, 10, 12, 14, 15, 16, 18, 19

SCORING RULES FOR SCALES,
19-ITEM DENTAL SATISFACTION QUESTIONNAIRE

Scale	Sum Scores for These Items (after scoring items as above)
Access	5 + 13 + 15
Availability/Convenience	7 + 9
Cost	3 + 10
Continuity	12
General Satisfaction	1
Pain Management	4 + 8 + 19
Quality	2 + 6 + 11 + 14 + 16 + 17 + 18
Access Total	3 + 5 + 7 + 9 + 10 + 13 + 15
Dental Satisfaction Index	1 + 2 + 3 + 4 + 5 + 6 + 7 + 8 + 9 + 10 + 11 + 12 + 13 + 14 + 15 + 16 + 17 + 18

NOTE: When items and scales are scored as indicated, higher scores indicate greater satisfaction.

Table B.2

SCORING RULES FOR ITEMS, 14-ITEM DENTAL SATISFACTION QUESTIONNAIRE

Scoring	Item No.
1 = Strongly agree 2 = Agree 3 = Not sure 4 = Disagree 5 = Strongly disagree	1, 3, 5, 8, 11, 13
5 = Strongly agree 4 = Agree 3 = Not sure 2 = Disagree 1 = Strongly disagree	2, 4, 6, 7, 9, 10, 12, 14

SCORING RULES FOR SCALES, 14-ITEM DENTAL SATISFACTION QUESTIONNAIRE

Scoring	Sum Scores for These Items (after scoring items as above)
Access	5 + 13
Availability/Convenience	7 + 9
Cost	3 + 10
Continuity	12
General Satisfaction	1
Pain Management	8
Quality	2 + 4 + 6 + 11 + 14
Access Total	3 + 5 + 7 + 9 + 10 + 13
Dental Satisfaction Index	1 + 2 + 3 + 4 + 5 + 6 + 7 + 8 + 9 + 10 + 11 + 12 + 13 + 14

NOTE: When items and scales are scored as indicated, higher scores indicate greater satisfaction. <u>Use of the 19-item questionnaire is recommended</u>; this information is included only to document the preliminary battery fielded in the HIE.

Appendix C

ITEMS USED TO MEASURE RESPONSE SET AND RESPONSE SET SCORING RULES

Table C.1

MATCHED PAIRS USED TO SCORE ACQUIESCENT AND OPPOSITION RESPONSE SETS

Pair Number	Item Number[a]	Item Content
1	16	There are enough family doctors around here
	42	There is a big shortage of family doctors around here
2	10	More hospitals are needed in this area
	38	There are enough hospitals in this area
3	21	I hardly ever see the same doctor when I go for medical care
	43	I see the same doctor just about every time I go for medical care
4	17	I think my doctor's office has everything needed to provide complete medical care
	28	My doctor's office lacks some things needed to provide complete medical care

NOTE: Each instance of incompatible agreements (choice of "strongly agree" or "agree") to both items in these pairs counted as an acquiescent response set pattern; each instance of incompatible disagreements (choice of "disagree" or "strongly disagree") to both items in any of these pairs counted as an opposition response set pattern. Scores on the ARS and the ORS measures could range from zero to four, and were computed separately for each respondent.

[a] Number refers to order of item placement in the 43-item Medical Care Satisfaction battery included in HIE Health Questionnaires.

Table C.2

Items and Scoring Rules for Social Desirability Response Set Measure

Item Content	Response Categories	Item Scoring
How often do you eat too much?	Very often, fairly often, sometimes, almost never	0
	Never	1
In general, would you say your morals have been above reproach?	Yes, definitely	1
	Yes, probably; I don't know; probably not, definitely not	0
How often have there been times in your life when you felt you acted like a coward?	Very often, fairly often, sometimes, almost never	0
	Never	1
Would you say that you give every penny you can to charity?	Yes, definitely; yes, for the most part	1
	Yes, I try; no	0
In choosing your friends, how important to you are things like their race, their religion, or their political beliefs?	Always very important, almost always important, usually important, not too important, hardly ever important	0
	Not important at all	1
If it is more convenient for you to do so, how often will you tell a lie?	Very often tell a lie, fairly often, sometimes tell a lie, almost never	0
	Never tell a lie	1
How often have you done anything of a sexual nature that society does not approve of?	Very often, fairly often, sometimes, almost never	0
	Never	1
Are your table manners at home just as good as they are when you are invited out to dinner?	Yes, always good	1
	Yes, with rare exceptions; yes, usually just as good; no, usually worse at home; no, quite a bit worse at home; no, very bad at home	0

NOTE: Socially Desirable Response Set (SDRS) was scored in two steps. First, item scores were summed after scoring as indicated above; scores for SDRS ranged from 0 to 8. Second, SDRS scores were recoded as follows: 8 = 6, 7 = 5, 6 = 4, 5 = 3, 4 = 2, 2 = 0, and 1 = 0. See Veit and Ware (forthcoming) for further details on the logic of scoring SDRS.

Appendix D

SUPPORTING TABLES

Table D.1

FREQUENCY DISTRIBUTIONS FOR RESPONSES TO DSQ ITEMS,
BY SITE AND ALL SITES COMBINED

Item	Abbreviated Content	Site[a]	Responses					Missing Responses
			1	2	3	4	5	
1	Dental care could be better	Day	9	103	92	142	18	2
		Seat	71	378	283	688	118	3
		Mass	30	270	205	502	63	1
		SC	8	73	94	93	12	0
		All	118	824	674	1425	211	6
2	Dentists check everything*	Day	3	43	86	214	18	2
		Seat	18	164	305	922	129	4
		Mass	5	116	204	657	88	1
		SC	3	25	79	155	18	0
		All	29	348	674	1948	253	7
3	Fees too high	Day	70	169	89	35	1	1
		Seat	302	661	392	165	18	3
		Mass	216	502	230	116	6	1
		SC	38	124	85	31	2	2
		All	626	1456	796	347	27	7
4	Avoid dentist because painful	Day	10	88	18	210	38	1
		Seat	87	285	53	891	222	5
		Mass	55	207	46	618	144	1
		SC	13	91	27	126	23	0
		All	165	671	144	1845	427	7
5	Wait long time in dentist's office	Day	22	113	54	167	8	2
		Seat	76	335	248	787	92	2
		Mass	50	244	144	583	49	1
		SC	15	83	67	110	5	0
		All	163	775	513	1647	154	5
6	Dentists treat patients with respect*	Day	2	37	86	219	20	2
		Seat	19	151	314	943	111	3
		Mass	9	98	182	690	91	1
		SC	0	14	82	162	22	1
		All	30	300	664	2014	244	7
7	Enough dentists around here*	Day	5	57	145	148	9	1
		Seat	13	107	521	802	95	2
		Mass	12	87	243	646	82	3
		SC	10	64	92	110	4	0
		All	40	315	1001	1706	190	6
8	Dentists should reduce pain	Day	18	134	119	89	4	1
		Seat	101	426	483	498	30	3
		Mass	90	337	294	327	22	1
		SC	18	103	107	49	3	0
		All	227	1000	1003	963	59	5

67

Table D.1—continued

Item	Abbreviated Content	Site[a]	Responses 1	2	3	4	5	Missing Responses
9	Dental care conveniently located*	Day	3	36	66	243	16	0
		Seat	11	99	225	1077	96	3
		Mass	7	98	106	779	80	2
		SC	5	49	61	152	13	0
		All	26	282	488	2551	205	5
10	Dentists avoid unnecessary expenses*	Day	22	130	166	44	2	1
		Seat	117	463	705	232	21	4
		Mass	61	323	516	156	14	1
		SC	14	68	158	36	4	0
		All	214	984	1545	468	41	6
11	Dentists not thorough	Day	4	62	144	145	9	1
		Seat	17	202	463	728	128	4
		Mass	14	160	321	531	44	0
		SC	2	46	125	102	5	0
		All	37	470	1053	1506	186	5
12	See same dentist*	Day	6	35	24	205	94	0
		Seat	28	121	48	884	457	2
		Mass	8	61	36	709	256	2
		SC	3	30	31	173	43	0
		All	45	247	139	1971	850	4
13	Hard to get appointment	Day	33	160	55	106	10	0
		Seat	157	621	155	491	114	2
		Mass	83	392	119	421	55	2
		SC	12	96	55	105	12	1
		All	285	1269	384	1123	191	5
14	Dentists relieve most problems*	Day	5	14	77	246	22	0
		Seat	10	58	187	1128	155	1
		Mass	3	36	143	806	82	1
		SC	0	13	61	190	16	0
		All	18	121	468	2370	275	2
15	Office hours good*	Day	8	72	80	195	9	0
		Seat	70	278	251	868	71	1
		Mass	23	176	162	662	47	0
		SC	4	28	71	161	16	0
		All	105	554	564	1886	143	1
16	Dentists explain what they do and cost*	Day	11	74	57	211	11	0
		Seat	74	329	181	839	115	1
		Mass	49	271	146	539	65	1
		SC	14	57	44	138	27	0
		All	148	731	428	1727	218	2

Table D.1—continued

Item	Abbreviated Content	Site[a]	Responses					Missing Responses
			1	2	3	4	5	
17	Keep people from problems with teeth	Day	12	121	147	82	2	1
		Seat	94	522	478	378	66	2
		Mass	56	412	321	268	13	0
		SC	23	98	107	45	7	0
		All	185	1153	1053	773	88	3
18	Dentist's offices modern*	Day	1	15	43	284	21	1
		Seat	6	55	227	1086	164	1
		Mass	0	38	190	752	90	1
		SC	2	10	69	170	29	0
		All	9	118	529	2292	304	3
19	Not concerned about pain*	Day	43	170	31	113	7	0
		Seat	314	615	75	454	80	2
		Mass	176	456	61	327	50	0
		SC	38	90	34	108	10	0
		All	571	1331	201	1002	147	2

NOTE: * denotes items that have been recoded so that scores indicate greater satisfaction (see App. B).

[a] Day = Dayton; Seat = Seattle, Washington; Mass = Fitchburg and Franklin County, Massachusetts; SC = Charleston and Georgetown County, South Carolina; All = All sites combined.

Table D.2

MEANS AND STANDARD DEVIATIONS, DSQ ITEMS, BY SITE

Item	Abbreviated Content	Dayton		Seattle		Massachusetts		South Carolina	
		Mean	S.D.	Mean	S.D.	Mean	S.D.	Mean	S.D.
1	Dental care could be better	3.16	0.97	3.26	1.06	3.28	1.00	3.10	0.93
2	Dentists check everything	3.55	0.79	3.64	0.83	3.66	0.80	3.57	0.79
3	Fees too high	2.25	0.88	2.31	0.94	2.25	0.92	2.41	0.88
4	Avoid dentist because painful	3.49	1.05	3.57	1.11	3.55	1.10	3.20	1.12
5	Wait long time at dentist's office	3.08	1.04	3.32	1.03	3.32	1.02	3.02	0.99
6	Dentists treat patient with respect	3.60	0.77	3.63	0.80	3.71	0.78	3.69	0.69
7	Enough dentists around here	3.27	0.80	3.56	0.75	3.65	0.78	3.12	0.90
8	Dentists could reduce pain	2.80	0.90	2.96	0.97	2.86	1.01	2.70	0.87
9	Dental care conveniently located	3.64	0.75	3.75	0.70	3.77	0.74	3.42	0.89
10	Dentists avoid unnecessary expenses	2.65	0.79	2.72	0.86	2.75	0.82	2.81	0.77
11	Dentists not thorough	3.26	0.80	3.49	0.86	3.40	0.84	3.22	0.76
12	See same dentist	3.95	0.92	4.05	0.90	4.07	0.75	3.80	0.86
13	Hard to get appointment	2.73	1.06	2.86	1.19	2.98	1.13	3.04	1.03
14	Dentists relieve most problems	3.73	0.69	3.89	0.65	3.87	0.59	3.75	0.63
15	Office hours good	3.34	0.90	3.38	0.98	3.50	0.89	3.56	0.80
16	Dentists explain what they do and cost	3.38	0.94	3.39	1.05	3.28	1.05	3.38	1.07
17	Keep people from problems with teeth	2.84	0.83	2.87	0.99	2.79	0.92	2.70	0.92
18	Dentists' offices modern	3.85	0.59	3.88	0.64	3.84	0.61	3.76	0.71
19	Not concerned about pain	2.65	1.10	2.59	1.25	2.64	1.20	2.86	1.17

Table D.3

CORRELATIONS BETWEEN DSQ ITEMS AND HYPOTHESIZED SUBSCALES, DAYTON (N = 364)

		Scale				
	Item Grouping/Item	ACCS	AVCO	COST	PAIN	QUAL
Access						
13	Hard to get appointment	37*	28	34	9	24
5	Wait long time at dentist's office	26*	28	33	23	37
15	Office hours good	21*	20	26	13	33
Availability/Convenience						
9	Dental care conveniently located	34	33*	24	17	35
7	Enough dentists around here	27	33*	19	15	27
Cost						
3	Fees too high	42	21	44*	4	30
10	Dentists avoid unnecessary expenses	35	24	44*	19	42
Pain						
8	Dentists should reduce pain	23	20	21	47*	39
4	Avoid dentist because painful	17	12	5	45*	24
19	Not concerned about pain	9	13	4	34*	15
Quality						
2	Dentists check everything	36	20	36	21	58*
11	Dentists not thorough	33	23	38	17	58*
16	Dentists explain what they do and cost	31	28	32	24	49*
6	Dentists treat patients with respect	28	28	28	20	47*
14	Dentists relieve most problems	25	19	10	19	40*
17	Keep people from problems with teeth	24	25	23	32	31*
18	Dentists' offices modern	20	24	11	14	39*

NOTE: * indicates item-scale correlation corrected for overlap; standard error of the correlation equals 0.05.

Table D.4

Correlations between DSQ Items and Hypothesized Subscales, Seattle (N = 1538)

Item Grouping/Item		Scale				
		ACCS	AVCO	COST	PAIN	QUAL
Access						
13	Hard to get appointment	38*	23	26	15	29
5	Wait long time at dentist's office	33*	27	29	22	35
15	Office hours good	28*	23	26	17	31
Availability/Convenience						
7	Enough dentists around here	29	38*	15	13	29
9	Dental care conveniently located	28	38*	14	14	28
Cost						
3	Fees too high	32	12	40*	19	24
10	Dentists avoid unnecessary expenses	32	16	40*	17	34
Pain						
8	Dentists should reduce pain	26	20	23	47*	30
4	Avoid dentist because painful	21	12	19	52*	23
19	Not concerned about pain	12	8	9	41*	15
Quality						
6	Dentists treat patients with respect	34	25	27	21	44*
11	Dentists not thorough	32	23	28	23	54*
2	Dentists check everything	28	25	22	18	56*
16	Dentists explain what they do and cost	27	17	23	11	32*
17	Keep people from problems with teeth	22	14	18	22	29*
18	Dentists' offices modern	21	25	9	14	35*
14	Dentists relieve most problems	17	18	8	7	28*
Unhypothesized						
1	Dental care could be better	37	26	33	31	53
12	See same dentist	29	24	17	17	32

NOTE: * indicates item-scale correlation corrected for overlap; standard error of the correlation equals 0.03.

Table D.5

CORRELATIONS BETWEEN DSQ ITEMS AND HYPOTHESIZED SUBSCALES, MASSACHUSETTS (N = 1070)

Item Grouping/Item		Scale				
		ACCS	AVCO	COST	PAIN	QUAL
Access						
13	Hard to get appointment	46*	26	31	25	31
5	Wait long time at dentist's office	40*	21	29	26	31
15	Office hours good	29*	23	19	13	28
Availability/Convenience						
9	Dental care conveniently located	34	36*	17	21	37
7	Enough dentists around here	19	36*	10	16	27
Cost						
3	Fees too high	32	9	41*	19	25
10	Dentists avoid unnecessary expenses	29	18	41*	11	32
Pain						
8	Dentists should reduce pain	28	21	17	52*	33
4	Avoid dentist because painful	26	19	12	53*	28
19	Not concerned about pain	17	12	14	41*	13
Quality						
11	Dentists not thorough	34	26	30	23	53*
6	Dentists treat patients with respect	28	33	28	24	45*
2	Dentists check everything	27	28	30	13	56*
14	Dentists relieve most problems	23	22	9	9	32*
17	Keep people from problems with teeth	23	15	22	24	27*
16	Dentists explain what they do and cost	20	15	15	17	34*
18	Dentists' offices modern	16	25	4	17	34*
Unhypothesized						
1	Dental care could be better	32	30	32	24	50
12	See same dentist	23	15	9	12	22

NOTE: * indicates item-scale correlation corrected for overlap; standard error of the correlation equals 0.03.

Table D.6

CORRELATIONS BETWEEN DSQ ITEMS AND HYPOTHESIZED SUBSCALES, SOUTH CAROLINA (N = 280)

Item Grouping/Item	ACCS	AVCO	COST	PAIN	QUAL
<u>Access</u>					
13 Hard to get appointment	40*	15	28	16	28
5 Wait long time at dentist's office	36*	35	26	20	38
15 Office hours good	25*	20	17	14	38
<u>Availability/Convenience</u>					
7 Enough dentists around here	31	45*	15	17	22
9 Dental care conveniently located	25	45*	15	17	28
<u>Cost</u>					
10 Dentists avoid unnecessary expenses	28	10	36*	5	27
3 Fees too high	27	19	36*	11	29
<u>Pain</u>					
4 Avoid dentist because painful	24	16	9	48*	32
8 Dentists should reduce pain	18	26	6	39*	26
19 Not concerned about pain	12	6	7	36*	18
<u>Quality</u>					
17 Keep people from problems with teeth	36	24	28	31	24*
6 Dentists treat patients with respect	32	16	11	14	29*
11 Dentists not thorough	31	32	29	29	57*
16 Dentists explain what they do and cost	27	11	19	13	32*
2 Dentists check everything	24	16	24	14	54*
18 Dentists' offices modern	24	11	9	22	45*
14 Dentists relieve most problems	19	11	6	16	26*
<u>Unhypothesized</u>					
1 Dental care could be better	31	16	31	23	51
12 See same dentist	18	13	11	14	31

NOTE: * indicates item-scale correlation corrected for overlap; standard error of the correlation equals 0.06.

Table D.7

CORRELATIONS BETWEEN DSQ ITEMS AND HYPOTHESIZED GLOBAL SCALES, DAYTON (N = 364)

		\multicolumn{4}{c}{Scale}			
\multicolumn{2}{l}{Item Grouping/Item}	ACCTOT	PAIN	QUAL	DSI
\multicolumn{6}{l}{Access Total}
3	Fees too high	46*	04	31	48*
10	Dentists avoid unnecessary expenses	45*	18	42	55*
13	Hard to get appointment	45*	09	24	45*
9	Dental care conveniently located	40*	17	35	49*
5	Wait long time at dentist's office	38*	23	37	55*
7	Enough dentists around here	32*	15	28	42*
15	Office hours good	30*	13	33	44*
\multicolumn{6}{l}{Pain}
8	Dentists should reduce pain	28	47*	39	55*
4	Avoid dentist because painful	16	45*	24	45*
19	Not concerned about pain	11	34*	15	32*
\multicolumn{6}{l}{Quality}
2	Dentists check everything	41	21	58*	61*
11	Dentists not thorough	42	17	58*	61*
16	Dentists explain what they do and cost	40	24	49*	57*
6	Dentists treat patients with respect	36	20	47*	53*
14	Dentists relieve most problems	25	19	40*	44*
18	Dentists' offices modern	24	14	39*	42*
17	Keep people from problems with teeth	31	32	31*	51*
\multicolumn{6}{l}{Unhypothesized}
1	Dental care could be better	38	26	50	59*
12	See same dentist	33	22	33	49*

NOTE: * indicates item-scale correlation corrected for overlap; standard error of the correlation equals 0.05.

Table D.8

CORRELATIONS BETWEEN DSQ ITEMS AND HYPOTHESIZED GLOBAL SCALES, SEATTLE (N = 1538)

Item Grouping/Item	ACCTOT	PAIN	QUAL	DSI
Access Total				
5 Wait long time at dentist's office	42*	22	35	46*
13 Hard to get appointment	41*	15	29	39*
10 Dentists avoid unnecessary expenses	39*	17	34	41*
3 Fees too high	37*	19	24	37*
15 Office hours good	36*	17	31	38*
7 Enough dentists around here	33*	13	29	35*
9 Dental care conveniently located	32*	14	28	35*
Pain				
4 Avoid dentist because painful	24	52*	23	38*
8 Dentists should reduce pain	31	47*	30	45*
19 Not concerned about pain	14	41*	15	24*
Quality				
2 Dentists check everything	34	18	55*	50*
11 Dentists not thorough	38	23	54*	54*
6 Dentists treat patients with respect	40	21	44*	48*
18 Dentists' offices modern	24	14	34*	33*
16 Dentists explain what they do and cost	31	11	32*	35*
17 Keep people from problems with teeth	25	22	29*	34*
14 Dentists relieve most problems	19	07	28*	26*
Unhypothesized				
1 Dental care could be better	44	31	53	57*
12 See same dentist	32	17	32	37*

NOTE: * indicates item-scale correlation corrected for overlap; standard error of the correlation equals 0.03.

Table D.9

Correlations between DSQ Items and Hypothesized Global Scales, Massachusetts (N = 1070)

Item Grouping/Item		Scale			
		ACCTOT	PAIN	QUAL	DSI
Access Total					
13	Hard to get appointment	49*	25	31	57*
5	Wait long time at dentist's office	43*	26	31	55*
9	Dental care conveniently located	38*	21	37	51*
10	Dentists avoid unnecessary expenses	38*	11	32	46*
3	Fees too high	36*	19	25	45*
15	Office hours good	33*	13	28	41*
7	Enough dentists around here	25*	16	27	39*
Pain					
4	Avoid dentist because painful	27	53*	28	52*
8	Dentists should reduce pain	32	52*	33	56*
19	Not concerned about pain	20	41*	13	39*
Quality					
2	Dentists check everything	38	13	56*	58*
11	Dentists not thorough	41	23	53*	61*
6	Dentists treat patients with respect	40	24	45*	56*
16	Dentists explain what they do and cost	24	17	34*	43*
18	Dentists' offices modern	20	17	34*	37*
14	Dentists relieve most problems	25	09	32*	37*
17	Keep people from problems with teeth	27	24	27*	44*
Unhypothesized					
1	Dental care could be better	43	24	50	61*
12	See same dentist	23	12	22	35*

NOTE: * indicates item-scale correlation corrected for overlap; standard error of the correlation equals 0.03.

Table D.10

CORRELATIONS BETWEEN DSQ ITEMS AND HYPOTHESIZED GLOBAL SCALES, SOUTH CAROLINA (N = 280)

		Scale			
	Item Grouping/Item	ACCTOT	PAIN	QUAL	DSI
Access Total					
5	Wait long time at dentist's office	47*	20	38	46*
7	Enough dentists around here	39*	17	22	34*
13	Hard to get appointment	38*	16	28	38*
3	Fees too high	35*	11	28	35*
9	Dental care conveniently located	35*	17	28	35*
10	Dentists avoid unnecessary expenses	32*	05	27	30*
15	Office hours good	29*	14	38	37*
Pain					
4	Avoid dentist because painful	24	48*	32	41*
8	Dentists should reduce pain	23	39*	26	36*
19	Not concerned about pain	11	36*	18	23*
Quality					
11	Dentists not thorough	42	29	57*	59*
2	Dentists check everything	29	14	54*	46*
18	Dentists' offices modern	22	22	45*	40*
16	Dentists explain what they do and cost	27	13	32*	32*
6	Dentists treat patients with respect	32	14	29*	36*
14	Dentists relieve most problems	18	16	26*	29*
17	Keep people from problems with teeth	41	31	24*	44*
Unhypothesized					
1	Dental care could be better	36	23	51	49*
12	See same dentist	20	14	31	29*

NOTE: * indicates item-scale correlation corrected for overlap; standard error of the correlation equals 0.06.

Table D.11

CUMULATIVE PERCENT OF VARIANCE EXPLAINED IN DSQ ITEMS[a]
BY ONE TO SIX PRINCIPAL COMPONENTS,
ALL SITES COMBINED

Item	Abbreviated Content	Number of Components					
		1	2	3	4	5	6
1	Dental care could be better	43	43	44	50	56	57
2	Dentists check everything	40	49	49	66	66	66
3	Fees too high	20	20	57	57	57	59
4	Avoid dentist because painful	20	58	63	63	63	66
5	Wait long time at dentist's office	31	31	33	38	44	50
6	Dentists treat patients with respect	33	35	35	36	40	42
7	Enough dentists around here	18	19	26	47	55	66
8	Dentists should reduce pain	26	61	63	63	64	64
9	Dental care conveniently located	23	24	31	50	54	64
10	Dentists avoid unnecessary expenses	23	24	50	50	55	55
11	Dentists not thorough	45	47	47	62	65	66
12	See same dentist	19	20	25	27	28	63
13	Hard to get appointment	24	24	31	47	47	50
14	Dentists relieve most problems	15	22	34	34	38	45
15	Office hours good	18	20	20	32	55	55
16	Dentists explain what they do and cost	19	22	22	23	38	43
17	Keep people from problems with teeth	19	23	24	28	34	43
18	Dentists' offices modern	18	23	41	42	47	47
19	Not concerned about pain	07	46	48	48	61	62
Percent of Total Variance[b]		24.1	31.9	39.0	45.1	50.5	55.5
Percent of Common Variance[c]		43.2	57.2	69.9	80.9	90.6	99.6

[a] Data are communality estimates for each item, or estimates of the variance in each item explained by the given number of factors.

[b] Calculated by dividing the sum of the eigenvalues for the given number of factors by 19, the number of items.

[c] Calculated by dividing the sum of the eigenvalues for the given number of factors by 4.612, the sum of the estimated item communalities (i.e., the estimate of common variance among the 19 items).

Table D.12

MEANS, STANDARD DEVIATIONS, AND SCALE MIDPOINTS,
DENTAL SATISFACTION MEASURES, BY SITE

Measure	Items	Dayton			Seattle			Massachusetts			South Carolina		
		Mean	S.D.	Prorated Mean[a]	Mean	S.D.	Prorated Mean	Mean	S.D.	Prorated Mean	Mean	S.D.	Prorated Mean
Access	3	9.15	2.08	61.0	9.56	2.29	63.7	9.79	2.24	65.3	9.62	2.03	64.1
Availability/ Convenience	2	6.91	1.27	69.1	7.30	1.20	73.0	7.43	1.25	74.3	6.55	1.52	65.5
Cost	2	4.92	1.43	49.2	5.03	1.51	50.3	5.00	1.46	50.0	5.23	1.37	52.3
Access Total	7	20.96	3.68	59.9	21.90	3.75	62.6	22.22	3.67	63.5	21.40	3.59	61.1
Pain Management	2	8.93	2.29	59.5	9.21	2.56	60.8	9.06	2.58	60.4	8.76	2.36	58.4
Quality	7	24.20	3.42	69.1	24.78	3.45	70.8	24.54	3.34	72.2	24.07	3.23	68.8
Continuity	1	3.95	0.92	79.0	4.05	0.90	81.0	4.07	0.75	81.4	3.80	0.86	76.0
General Satisfaction	1	3.16	0.97	63.2	3.26	1.06	65.2	3.28	1.00	65.5	3.10	0.93	62.0
Dental Satisfaction Index	19	61.22	8.26	64.4	63.11	8.54	66.4	63.17	8.24	66.5	61.12	7.91	64.3

[a] Prorated mean = raw mean expressed as a percentage of highest possible scale score, which equals 5 times the number of items.

Table D.13

FREQUENCY DISTRIBUTIONS FOR ACCESS SCALE, BY SITE

Score	All Sites f	%	Dayton f	%	Seattle f	%	Massachusetts f	%	South Carolina f	%
3	15	0.5	1	0.3	10	0.7	4	0.4	0	0.0
4	39	1.2	5	1.4	15	1.0	19	1.8	0	0.0
5	67	2.1	9	2.5	34	2.2	21	2.0	3	1.1
6	173	5.4	24	6.7	88	5.8	48	4.5	13	4.7
7	240	7.5	31	8.7	129	8.5	52	4.9	28	10.1
8	514	16.0	70	19.7	237	15.6	161	15.2	46	16.7
9	411	12.8	55	15.4	195	12.8	123	11.6	38	13.8
10	654	20.4	74	20.8	302	19.9	222	21.0	56	20.3
11	276	8.6	30	8.4	129	8.5	97	9.2	20	7.2
12	609	19.0	48	13.5	255	16.8	246	23.2	60	21.7
13	137	4.3	4	1.1	86	5.7	39	3.7	8	2.9
14	49	1.5	2	0.6	28	1.8	16	1.5	3	1.1
15	27	0.8	3	0.8	12	0.8	11	1.0	1	0.4

NOTE: Calculations of percentages do not take missing scores into account.

Table D.14

FREQUENCY DISTRIBUTIONS FOR AVAILABILITY/CONVENIENCE SCALE, BY SITE

Score	All Sites f	%	Dayton f	%	Seattle f	%	Massachusetts f	%	South Carolina f	%
2	13	0.4	1	0.3	5	0.3	3	0.3	4	1.4
3	15	0.5	2	0.6	4	0.3	5	0.5	4	1.4
4	104	3.2	18	5.1	31	2.0	26	2.5	29	10.5
5	140	4.4	17	4.8	62	4.1	37	3.5	24	8.7
6	553	17.2	82	23.0	255	16.8	156	14.7	60	21.7
7	684	21.3	94	26.4	346	22.8	188	17.8	56	20.3
8	1480	46.1	133	37.4	709	46.6	543	51.3	95	34.4
9	128	4.0	4	1.1	63	4.1	59	5.6	2	0.7
10	94	2.9	5	1.4	45	3.0	42	4.0	2	0.7

NOTE: Calculations of percentages do not take missing scores into account.

Table D.15

FREQUENCY DISTRIBUTIONS FOR COST SCALE, BY SITE

Score	All Sites f	All Sites %	Dayton f	Dayton %	Seattle f	Seattle %	Massachusetts f	Massachusetts %	South Carolina f	South Carolina %
3	69	2.1	5	1.4	38	2.5	24	2.3	2	0.7
4	87	2.7	7	2.0	39	2.6	34	3.2	7	2.5
5	160	5.0	13	3.7	79	5.2	45	4.2	23	8.3
6	258	8.0	39	11.0	107	7.0	89	8.4	23	8.3
7	240	7.5	26	7.3	112	7.4	76	7.2	26	9.4
8	440	13.7	59	16.6	197	13.0	143	13.5	41	14.9
9	463	14.4	50	14.0	226	14.9	144	13.6	43	15.6
10	532	16.6	68	19.1	245	16.1	179	16.9	40	14.5
11	359	11.2	37	10.4	168	11.1	121	11.4	33	12.0
12	419	13.0	38	10.7	214	14.1	137	12.9	30	10.9
13	118	3.7	13	3.7	59	3.9	40	3.8	6	2.2
14	46	1.4	1	0.3	23	1.5	21	2.0	1	0.4
15	20	0.6	0	0.0	13	0.9	6	0.6	1	0.4

NOTE: Calculations of percentages do not take missing scores into account.

Table D.16

FREQUENCY DISTRIBUTIONS FOR PAIN SCALE, BY SITE

Score	All Sites f	All Sites %	Dayton f	Dayton %	Seattle f	Seattle %	Massachusetts f	Massachusetts %	South Carolina f	South Carolina %
2	146	4.5	17	4.8	78	5.1	45	4.2	6	2.2
3	311	9.7	37	10.4	148	9.7	105	9.9	21	7.6
4	747	23.3	91	25.6	341	22.4	256	24.2	59	21.4
5	774	24.1	82	23.0	370	24.3	260	24.6	62	22.5
6	802	25.0	91	25.6	369	24.3	251	23.7	91	33.0
7	245	7.6	21	5.9	114	7.5	86	8.1	24	8.7
8	161	5.0	16	4.5	86	5.7	48	4.5	11	4.0
9	21	0.7	1	0.3	10	0.7	8	0.8	2	0.7
10	4	0.1	0	0.0	4	0.3	0	0.0	0	0.0

NOTE: Calculations of percentages do not take missing scores into account.

Table D.17

FREQUENCY DISTRIBUTIONS FOR QUALITY SCALE, BY SITE

Score	All Sites f	All Sites %	Dayton f	Dayton %	Seattle f	Seattle %	Massachusetts f	Massachusetts %	South Carolina f	South Carolina %
7	0	0.0	0	0.0	0	0.0	0	0.0	0	0.0
8	1	0.0	1	0.3	0	0.0	0	0.0	0	0.0
9	0	0.0	0	0.0	0	0.0	0	0.0	0	0.0
10	0	0.0	0	0.0	0	0.0	0	0.0	0	0.0
11	1	0.0	0	0.0	1	0.1	0	0.0	0	0.0
12	1	0.0	0	0.0	1	0.1	0	0.0	0	0.0
13	5	0.2	1	0.3	3	0.2	1	0.1	0	0.0
14	6	0.2	1	0.3	3	0.2	2	0.2	0	0.0
15	11	0.3	2	0.6	6	0.4	1	0.1	2	0.7
16	29	0.9	6	1.7	11	0.7	10	0.9	2	0.7
17	35	1.1	3	0.8	12	0.8	14	1.3	6	2.2
18	66	2.1	10	2.8	25	1.6	24	2.3	7	2.5
19	84	2.6	8	2.2	38	2.5	29	2.7	9	3.3
20	125	3.9	11	3.1	61	4.0	45	4.2	8	2.9
21	197	6.1	23	6.5	90	5.9	64	6.0	20	7.2
22	241	7.5	21	5.9	122	8.0	75	7.1	23	8.3
23	302	9.4	35	9.8	133	8.7	98	9.3	36	13.0
24	381	11.9	56	15.7	155	10.2	129	12.2	41	14.9
25	363	11.3	43	12.1	164	10.8	124	11.7	32	11.6
26	454	14.1	51	14.3	214	14.1	158	14.9	31	11.2
27	341	10.6	29	8.1	185	12.2	101	9.5	26	9.4
28	277	8.6	35	9.8	130	8.6	98	9.3	14	5.1
29	116	3.6	10	2.8	60	3.9	37	3.5	9	3.3
30	65	2.0	2	0.6	47	3.1	13	1.2	3	1.1
31	51	1.6	3	0.8	29	1.9	16	1.5	3	1.1
32	24	0.7	2	0.6	11	0.7	8	0.8	3	1.1
33	11	0.3	1	0.3	6	0.4	4	0.4	0	0.0
34	16	0.5	2	0.6	9	0.6	4	0.4	1	0.4
35	8	0.2	0	0.0	4	0.3	4	0.4	0	0.0

NOTE: Calculations of percentages do not take missing scores into account.

Table D.18

FREQUENCY DISTRIBUTIONS FOR ACCESS TOTAL SCALE, BY SITE

Score	All Sites f	All Sites %	Dayton f	Dayton %	Seattle f	Seattle %	Massachusetts f	Massachusetts %	South Carolina f	South Carolina %
7	3	0.1	1	0.3	2	0.1	0	0.0	0	0.0
8	0	0.0	0	0.0	0	0.0	0	0.0	0	0.0
9	1	0.0	0	0.0	0	0.0	1	0.1	0	0.0
10	6	0.2	1	0.3	4	0.3	1	0.1	0	0.0
11	13	0.4	1	0.3	6	0.4	4	0.4	2	0.7
12	13	0.4	3	0.8	3	0.2	6	0.6	1	0.4
13	28	0.9	5	1.4	12	0.8	9	0.8	2	0.7
14	36	1.1	7	2.0	13	0.9	10	0.9	6	2.2
15	56	1.7	9	2.5	26	1.7	18	1.7	3	1.1
16	101	3.1	14	3.9	45	3.0	29	2.7	13	4.7
17	127	4.0	17	4.8	58	3.8	40	3.8	12	4.3
18	176	5.5	23	6.5	104	6.8	36	3.4	13	4.7
19	226	7.0	33	9.3	110	7.2	59	5.6	24	8.7
20	303	9.4	35	9.8	143	9.4	94	8.9	31	11.2
21	352	11.0	48	13.5	163	10.7	104	9.8	37	13.4
22	363	11.3	35	9.8	159	10.5	144	13.6	25	9.1
23	306	9.5	33	9.3	155	10.2	92	8.7	26	9.4
24	317	9.9	33	9.3	155	10.2	105	9.9	24	8.7
25	277	8.6	24	6.7	114	7.5	122	11.5	17	6.2
26	212	6.6	11	3.1	97	6.4	84	7.9	20	7.2
27	130	4.0	10	2.8	63	4.1	45	4.2	12	4.3
28	83	2.6	11	3.1	39	2.6	27	2.5	6	2.2
29	31	1.0	0	0.0	18	1.2	11	1.0	2	0.7
30	25	0.8	2	0.6	14	0.9	9	0.8	0	0.0
31	10	0.3	0	0.0	6	0.4	4	0.4	0	0.0
32	9	0.3	0	0.0	7	0.5	2	0.2	0	0.0
33	2	0.1	0	0.0	0	0.0	2	0.2	0	0.0
34	4	0.1	0	0.0	3	0.2	1	0.1	0	0.0
35	1	0.0	0	0.0	1	0.1	0	0.0	0	0.0

NOTE: Calculations of percentages do not take missing scores into account.

Table D.19

FREQUENCY DISTRIBUTIONS FOR DENTAL SATISFACTION INDEX SCALE, BY SITE

Score	All Sites f	%	Dayton f	%	Seattle f	%	Massachusetts f	%	South Carolina f	%
19	0	0.0	0	0.0	0	0.0	0	0.0	0	0.0
20	0	0.0	0	0.0	0	0.0	0	0.0	0	0.0
21	0	0.0	0	0.0	0	0.0	0	0.0	0	0.0
22	0	0.0	0	0.0	0	0.0	0	0.0	0	0.0
23	0	0.0	0	0.0	0	0.0	0	0.0	0	0.0
24	0	0.0	0	0.0	0	0.0	0	0.0	0	0.0
25	0	0.0	0	0.0	0	0.0	0	0.0	0	0.0
26	0	0.0	0	0.0	0	0.0	0	0.0	0	0.0
27	0	0.0	0	0.0	0	0.0	0	0.0	0	0.0
28	0	0.0	0	0.0	0	0.0	0	0.0	0	0.0
29	0	0.0	0	0.0	0	0.0	0	0.0	0	0.0
30	2	0.1	2	0.6	0	0.0	0	0.0	0	0.0
31	0	0.0	0	0.0	0	0.0	0	0.0	0	0.0
32	1	0.0	0	0.0	1	0.1	0	0.0	0	0.0
33	1	0.0	0	0.0	1	0.1	0	0.0	0	0.0
34	1	0.0	0	0.0	1	0.1	0	0.0	0	0.0
35	1	0.0	0	0.0	1	0.1	0	0.0	0	0.0
36	3	0.1	1	0.3	0	0.0	2	0.2	0	0.0
37	1	0.0	0	0.0	0	0.0	0	0.0	1	0.4
38	4	0.1	0	0.0	1	0.1	2	0.2	0	0.0
39	4	0.1	2	0.6	1	0.1	0	0.0	1	0.4
40	5	0.2	0	0.0	3	0.2	2	0.2	0	0.0
41	7	0.2	0	0.0	3	0.2	4	0.4	0	0.0
42	11	0.3	2	0.6	6	0.4	2	0.2	1	0.4
43	7	0.2	1	0.3	2	0.1	4	0.4	0	0.0
44	14	0.4	1	0.3	8	0.5	3	0.3	2	0.7
45	18	0.6	2	0.6	8	0.5	7	0.7	1	0.4
46	21	0.7	1	0.3	8	0.5	11	1.0	1	0.4
47	33	1.0	9	2.5	16	1.1	5	0.5	3	1.1
48	39	1.2	7	2.0	13	0.9	11	1.0	8	2.9
49	25	0.8	2	0.6	11	0.7	10	0.9	2	0.7
50	56	1.7	6	1.7	29	1.9	12	1.1	9	3.3
51	38	1.2	5	1.4	20	1.3	9	0.8	4	1.4
52	55	1.7	10	2.8	24	1.6	18	1.7	3	1.1
53	72	2.2	9	2.5	38	2.5	22	2.1	3	1.1
54	65	2.0	8	2.2	28	1.8	23	2.2	6	2.2
55	96	3.0	11	3.1	49	3.2	25	2.4	11	4.0
56	117	3.6	10	2.8	51	3.4	41	3.9	15	5.4
57	131	4.1	16	4.5	57	3.7	32	3.0	26	9.4
58	121	3.8	16	4.5	47	3.1	49	4.6	9	3.3
59	135	4.2	16	4.5	67	4.4	39	3.7	13	4.7
60	154	4.8	16	4.5	73	4.8	46	4.3	19	6.9

Table D.19—continued

Score	All Sites f	%	Dayton f	%	Seattle f	%	Massachusetts f	%	South Carolina f	%
61	121	3.8	15	4.2	52	3.4	40	3.8	14	5.1
62	145	4.5	19	5.3	67	4.4	47	4.4	12	4.3
63	157	4.9	15	4.2	79	5.2	49	4.6	14	5.1
64	170	5.3	24	6.7	83	5.5	52	4.9	11	4.0
65	166	5.2	26	7.3	74	4.9	55	5.2	11	4.0
66	131	4.1	13	3.7	58	3.8	51	4.8	9	3.3
67	140	4.4	8	2.2	75	4.9	48	4.5	9	3.3
68	171	5.3	24	6.7	65	4.3	73	6.9	9	3.3
69	138	4.3	14	3.9	75	4.9	44	4.2	5	1.8
70	119	3.7	7	2.0	63	4.1	44	4.2	5	1.8
71	92	2.9	9	2.5	41	2.7	32	3.0	10	3.6
72	83	2.6	10	2.8	39	2.6	26	2.5	8	2.9
73	73	2.3	3	0.8	34	2.2	31	2.9	5	1.8
74	52	1.6	4	1.1	25	1.6	18	1.7	5	1.8
75	43	1.3	2	0.6	20	1.3	20	1.9	1	0.4
76	33	1.0	1	0.3	13	0.9	17	1.6	2	0.7
77	21	0.7	1	0.3	11	0.7	7	0.7	2	0.7
78	28	0.9	2	0.6	22	1.4	3	0.3	1	0.4
79	18	0.6	0	0.0	12	0.8	3	0.3	3	1.1
80	15	0.5	0	0.0	13	0.9	2	0.2	0	0.0
81	7	0.2	3	0.8	4	0.3	0	0.0	0	0.0
82	9	0.3	1	0.3	7	0.5	0	0.0	1	0.4
83	11	0.3	0	0.0	6	0.4	5	0.5	0	0.0
84	4	0.1	0	0.0	1	0.1	2	0.2	1	0.4
85	8	0.2	0	0.0	4	0.3	4	0.4	0	0.0
86	9	0.3	2	0.6	4	0.3	3	0.3	0	0.0
87	2	0.1	0	0.0	1	0.1	1	0.1	0	0.0
88	1	0.0	0	0.0	1	0.1	0	0.0	0	0.0
89	3	0.1	0	0.0	2	0.1	1	0.1	0	0.0
90	1	0.0	0	0.0	0	0.0	1	0.1	0	0.0
91	0	0.0	0	0.0	0	0.0	0	0.0	0	0.0
92	1	0.0	0	0.0	0	0.0	1	0.1	0	0.0
93	1	0.0	0	0.0	1	0.1	0	0.0	0	0.0

NOTE: Calculations of percentages do not take missing scores into account.

Table D.20

COMPARISON BETWEEN RATINGS OF DENTAL AND MEDICAL CARE ON MATCHED QUESTIONNAIRE ITEMS, DAYTON

Abbreviated Item Content[a]	Rating[b] Dental	Rating[b] Medical	Mean Difference	t
Accessibility				
Keeps patients waiting	3.08 (1.05)	2.39 (0.96)	0.68	10.99**
Fees too high	2.25 (0.89)	2.21 (0.91)	0.05	1.07
Convenient places	3.64 (0.75)	3.46 (0.86)	0.22	4.57**
Hard to get appointments	2.72 (1.06)	3.08 (1.05)	-0.37	-5.67**
Office hours good	3.35 (0.90)	3.24 (0.97)	0.10	2.52*
Continuity				
See same provider	3.95 (0.92)	3.89 (0.82)	0.06	1.01
Quality				
Checks everything	3.55 (0.80)	2.78 (0.87)	0.77	14.43**
Not thorough enough	3.26 (0.80)	2.86 (0.92)	0.41	6.57**
Treats patients with respect	3.60 (0.77)	3.32 (0.90)	0.27	6.33**
General Satisfaction				
Care could be better	3.16 (1.00)	2.73 (0.84)	0.43	7.32**

NOTE: N ranged from 361 to 363 because of missing data.

[a] Items differ only in reference to dental or medical care/dentist or doctor.

[b] Mean score with standard deviation in parentheses; higher score indicates more favorable rating.

*$p < 0.01$.

**$p < 0.001$, two-tailed test of significance of mean difference.

Table D.21

COMPARISON BETWEEN RATINGS OF DENTAL AND MEDICAL CARE ON MATCHED QUESTIONNAIRE ITEMS, SEATTLE

Abbreviated Item Content[a]	Rating[b] Dental	Medical	Mean Difference	t
Accessibility				
Keeps patients waiting	3.32 (1.03)	2.50 (1.06)	0.81	25.32**
Fees too high	2.31 (0.94)	2.32 (0.98)	-0.01	-0.72
Convenient places	3.74 (0.70)	3.44 (0.88)	0.30	12.64**
Hard to get appointments	2.86 (1.19)	2.92 (1.14)	-0.06	-1.67
Office hours good	3.38 (0.98)	3.21 (0.98)	0.17	7.69**
Continuity				
See same provider	4.05 (0.90)	3.63 (0.98)	0.42	14.08**
Quality				
Checks everything	3.64 (0.83)	2.75 (0.92)	0.89	31.69**
Not thorough enough	3.49 (0.86)	2.96 (1.03)	0.53	17.34**
Treats patients with respect	3.63 (0.80)	3.26 (0.94)	0.37	14.36**
General Satisfaction				
Care could be better	3.26 (1.06)	2.73 (0.92)	0.53	17.24**

NOTE: N ranged from 1526 to 1533 because of missing data.

[a] Items differ only in reference to dental or medical care/dentist or doctor.

[b] Mean score with standard deviation in parentheses; higher score indicates more favorable rating.

** $p < 0.001$, two-tailed test of significance of mean difference.

Table D.22

COMPARISON BETWEEN RATINGS OF DENTAL AND MEDICAL CARE ON MATCHED QUESTIONNAIRE ITEMS, MASSACHUSETTS

Abbreviated Item Content[a]	Rating[b] Dental	Rating[b] Medical	Mean Difference	t
Accessibility				
Keeps patients waiting	3.32 (1.02)	2.57 (1.01)	0.80	21.59**
Fees too high	2.25 (0.92)	2.24 (0.96)	0.01	0.12
Convenient places	3.77 (0.74)	3.59 (0.85)	0.18	6.85**
Hard to get appointments	2.97 (1.13)	2.91 (1.08)	0.06	1.62
Office hours good	3.50 (0.89)	3.25 (0.94)	0.25	8.39**
Continuity				
See same provider	4.07 (0.75)	3.76 (0.85)	0.31	9.55
Quality				
Checks everything	3.66 (0.80)	2.97 (0.93)	0.69	21.43**
Not thorough enough	3.41 (0.84)	3.03 (1.02)	0.38	10.87**
Treats patients with respect	3.71 (0.78)	3.37 (0.96)	0.34	11.76**
General Satisfaction				
Care could be better	3.28 (1.00)	2.84 (0.93)	0.44	12.11**

NOTE: N ranged from 1064 to 1068 because of missing data.

[a] Items differ only in reference to dental or medical care/dentist or doctor.

[b] Mean score with standard deviation in parentheses; higher score indicates more favorable rating.

** $p < 0.001$, two-tailed test of significance of mean difference.

Table D.23

COMPARISON BETWEEN RATINGS OF DENTAL AND MEDICAL CARE
ON MATCHED QUESTIONNAIRE ITEMS, SOUTH CAROLINA

Abbreviated Item Content[a]	Rating[b] Dental	Medical	Mean Difference	t
Accessibility				
Keeps patients waiting	3.02 (0.99)	2.10 (0.91)	0.92	12.16**
Fees too high	2.41 (0.89)	2.35 (0.97)	0.06	1.00
Convenient places	3.43 (0.88)	3.24 (0.98)	0.19	3.02*
Hard to get appointments	3.03 (1.03)	2.65 (0.98)	0.37	4.71**
Office hours good	3.56 (0.80)	3.21 (0.93)	0.35	5.91*
Continuity				
See same provider	3.80 (0.87)	3.65 (1.00)	0.14	2.18*
Quality				
Checks everything	3.58 (0.78)	2.92 (0.92)	0.66	10.36**
Not thorough enough	3.21 (0.76)	2.81 (0.96)	0.40	5.92**
Treats patients with respect	3.68 (0.69)	3.42 (0.91)	0.26	4.89**
General Satisfaction				
Care could be better	3.11 (0.93)	2.76 (0.83)	0.35	5.46**

NOTE: N ranged from 277 to 280 because of missing data.

[a] Items differ only in reference to dental or medical care/dentist or doctor.

[b] Mean score with standard deviation in parentheses; higher score indicates more favorable rating.

*$p < 0.01$.

**$p < 0.001$, two-tailed test of significance of mean difference.

Appendix E

RECOMMENDED ADDITIONS TO DENTAL SATISFACTION QUESTIONNAIRE TO MEASURE INTERPERSONAL ASPECTS OF DENTAL CARE

Dentists always do their best to keep the patient from worrying.

Sometimes dentists act rude toward their patients.

Dentists treat their patients in a friendly manner.

REFERENCES

Bailit, H.L., and M.N. Raskin, "Assessing Quality of Care and Oral Health in a Population With Dental Insurance," *Inquiry* 15:359-370, 1978.

Becker, M.H., R.H. Drachman, and J.P. Kirscht, "A Field Experiment To Evaluate Various Outcomes of Continuity of Physician Care," *American Journal of Public Health* 64:1062, 1974.

Belok, G., "Attitudes toward a Dental Program at the Yale Health Plan," *Journal of the American College Health Association* 25:322-326, 1977.

Bene, A.A., W.E. Novasky, and S.G. Geldart, "Public Attitudes, Utilization Patterns and Socio-economic Determinants," *Journal of the Canadian Dental Association* 40:444-451, 1974.

Bernstein, D.A., R.A. Kleinknecht, and L.D. Alexander, "Antecedents of Dental Fear," *Journal of Public Health Dentistry* 39:112-124, 1979.

Biro, P.A., and N.D. Hewson, "A Survey of Patients' Attitudes to Their Dentists," *Australian Dental Journal* 21:338-394, 1976.

Blum, S., and R.W. Tuthill, "An Epidemiologic Analysis of the Use of Dental Services and of Attitudes of Students at a Major University," *Journal of the American College Health Association* 25:327-330, 1977.

Breslau, N., and K.G. Reeb, "Continuity of Care in a University-based Practice," *Journal of Medical Education* 50:965-969, 1975.

Campbell, D.T., and D.W. Fiske, "Convergent and Discriminant Validation by the Multitrait-Multimethod Matrix," *Psychological Bulletin* 56:81-105, 1959.

Cattell, R.B., ed., *Handbook of Multivariate Experimental Psychology,* Chicago, Rand McNally and Company, 1966.

Clark, J.D., and J.C. Morton, "Behavioral Assessment: An Appraisal of Beliefs and Behaviors Related to Treatment," *Dental Clinics of North America* 21:515-530, 1977.

Collett, H.A., "Influence of Dentist-Patient Relationship on Attitudes and Adjustment to Dental Treatment," *Journal of the American Dental Association* 79:879-884, 1969.

Comrey, A.L., *Comrey Personality Scales,* San Diego, Testing Services, 1970.

Cronbach, L.J., "Coefficient Alpha and the Internal Structure of Tests," *Psychometrika* 16:297-334, 1951.

Davies, A.R., and J.E. Ware, Jr., *Measuring Health Perceptions in the Health Insurance Experiment,* The Rand Corporation, R-2711-HHS, 1981.

Fanning, E.A., and P.I. Leppard, "A Survey of University Students in South Australia, Part III: Attitudes to Dental Treatment," *Australian Dental Journal* 18:20-22, 1973.

Guertin, W.H., and J.P. Bailey, Jr., *Introduction to Modern Factor Analysis,* Ann Arbor, Edwards Brothers, Inc., 1970.

Helmstadter, G.C., *Principles of Psychological Measurement,* New York, Appleton-Century-Crofts, 1964.

Hengst, A., and K. Roghmann, "The Two Dimensions in Satisfaction with Dental Care," *Medical Care* 16:202-213, 1978.

Howard, K.I., and G.G. Forehand, "A Method for Correcting Item-Total Correlations for the Effect of Relevant-Item Inclusion," *Educational and Psychological Measurement* 22:731-735, 1962.

Hulka, B.C., S.J. Zyzanski, J.C. Cassel, and S.J. Thompson, "Scale for the Measurement of Attitudes Toward Physicians and Primary Medical Care," *Medical Care* 8:429-436, 1970.

Jenny, J., J.P. Frazier, R.A. Bagramian, and J.M. Proshek, "Parents' Satisfaction and Dissatisfaction with Their Children's Dentist," *Journal of Public Health Dentistry* 33:211-221, 1973.

Kasteller, J., R.L. Kane, D.M. Olsen, et al., "Issues Underlying Prevalence of 'Doctor-shopping' Behavior," *Journal of Health and Social Behavior* 17:328-339, 1976.

Koslowsky, M., H. Bailit, and P. Valluzzo, "Satisfaction of the Patient and the Provider; Evaluation by Questionnaire," *Journal of Public Health Dentistry* 34:188-194, 1974.

Kriesberg, L., and B.R. Treiman, "Dentists and the Practice of Dentistry as Viewed by the Public," *Journal of the American Dental Association* 64:806-821, 1962.

Lengkeek, R., C.J. Maas-De Wall, M.A. Van Groenestijn, P.A. Mileman, and J.N. Swallow, "Patient Evaluation of Dental Treatment," *British Dental Journal* 146:343-345, 1979.

Likert, R., "A Technique for the Measurement of Attitudes," *Archives of Psychology* 140:1-55, 1932.

Marquis, M.S., A.R. Davies, and J.E. Ware, Jr., "Patient Satisfaction and Change in Medical Care Provider: A Longitudinal Study," *Medical Care*, in press.

McKeithen, E.J., "The Patient's Image of the Dentist," *Journal of the American College of Dentistry* 33:87-107, 1966.

Messick, S., "Separate Set and Content Scores for Personality and Attitude Scales," *Educational and Psychological Measurement* 21:915-923, 1961.

Murray, B.P., and H.J. Wiese, "Satisfaction with Care and the Utilization of Dental Services at a Neighborhood Health Center," *Journal of Public Health Dentistry* 35:170-176, 1975.

Newhouse, J.P., "A Design for a Health Insurance Study," *Inquiry* 11:5-27, 1974.

Richards, N.D., "Utilization of Dental Services," in N.D. Richards and L.K. Cohen, eds., *Social Sciences and Dentistry: A Critical Bibliography,* The Hague, A. Sijthoff, 1971, pp. 209-240.

Richards, N.D., A.J. Willcocks, J.A. Bulman, and G.I. Slack, "A Survey of Dental Health and Attitudes Towards Dentistry in Two Communities: Part I, Sociological Data," *British Dental Journal* 118:199-205, 1965.

Rogers, W.H., K.N. Williams, and R.H. Brook, *Conceptualization and Measurement of Health for Adults in the Health Insurance Study: Vol. VII, Power Analysis of Health Status Measures,* The Rand Corporation, R-1987/7-HEW, 1979.

Scarrott, D.M., "Attitudes to Dentists," *British Dental Journal* 127:583-590, 1969.

Shortell, S.M., "Continuity of Care: Conceptualization and Measurement," *Medical Care* 14:377-391, 1976.

Shortell, S.M., W.C. Richardson, J.P. LoGerfo, et al., "The Relationship among Dimensions of Health Services in Two Provider Systems: A Causal Model Approach," *Journal of Health and Social Behavior* 18:139-159, 1977.

Smith, L.H., G.A. Goldberg, R.H. Brook, et al., *The Health Insurance Study Screening Examination Procedures Manual,* The Rand Corporation, R-2101-HEW, 1978.

Snyder, M.K., and J.E. Ware, Jr., *A Study of Twenty-Two Hypothesized Dimensions of Patient Attitudes Regarding Medical Care,* NTIS Publ. No. PB-239-518/AS, Springfield, Va., National Technical Information Service, 1974.

Stacey, D.C., B.A. Slome, and D. Musgrave, "Factors Affecting Patient Completion of Treatment within a Student Dental Clinic," *Journal of Dental Education* 42:609-617, 1978.

Strauss, R.P., "Sociocultural Influences upon Preventive Health Behavior and Attitudes Towards Dentistry," *American Journal of Public Health* 66:375-377, 1976.

Sword, R.O., "Psychological Aspects of the Doctor-Patient Relationship," *Journal of the Colorado Dental Association*, pp. 33-35, August 1969.

Thurstone, L.L., and E.J. Chave, *The Measurement of Attitude,* Chicago, University of Chicago Press, 1929.

U.S. Department of Health, Education, and Welfare, "Current Estimates from the Health Interview Survey: United States—1978," DHEW Publ. No. (PHS) 80-1551, U.S. Government Printing Office, Washington, D.C., 1979.

Veit, C., and J.E. Ware, Jr., *Refinements in the Measurement of Mental Health for Adults in the Health Insurance Study,* The Rand Corporation, R-2737-HHS, forthcoming.

Ware, J.E., Jr., "Some Issues in the Measurement of Patient Satisfaction with Health Care Services," The Rand Corporation, P-6021, 1977.

Ware, J.E., Jr., "Effects of Acquiescent Response Set on Patient Satisfaction Ratings," *Medical Care* 16:327-336, 1978.

Ware, J.E., Jr., R.H. Brook, A. Davies-Avery, et al., *Conceptualization and Measurement of Health for Adults in the Health Insurance Study: Vol. I, Model of Health and Methodology,* The Rand Corporation, R-1987/1-HEW, 1980.

Ware, J.E., Jr., A. Davies-Avery, and A.L. Stewart, "The Measurement and Meaning of Patient Satisfaction," *Health and Medical Care Services Review* 1:1-15, 1978.

Ware, J.E., Jr., R.L. Kane, A.R. Davies, and R.H. Brook, *An Experimental Approach to Validating Patients' Quality of Care Assessments,* The Rand Corporation, forthcoming.

Ware, J.E., Jr., W.G. Miller, and M.K. Snyder, *Comparison of Factor Analytic Methods in the Development of Health-Related Indexes from Questionnaire Data,* NTIS Publ. No. PB-239-517/AS, Springfield, Va., National Technical Information Service, 1973.

Ware, J.E., Jr., M.K. Snyder, and W.R. Wright, *Development and Validation of Scales to Measure Patient Satisfaction with Health Care Services, Volume 1 of a Final Report, Part A: Review of Literature, Overview of Methods and Results Regarding Construction of Scales,* NTIS Publ. No. PB 288-329, Springfield, Va., National Technical Information Service, 1976.

Ware, J.E., Jr., W.R. Wright, M.K. Snyder, and G.C. Chu, "Consumer Perceptions of Health Care Services: Implications for Academic Medicine," *Journal of Medical Education* 50: 839-848, 1975.

Weinstein, P., P. Milgrom, P. Ratener, W. Read, and K. Morrison, "Dentists' Perceptions of Their Patients: Relation to Quality of Care," *Journal of Public Health Dentistry* 38:10-21, 1978.

Winkler, J.D., D.E. Kanouse, and J.E. Ware, Jr., "Controlling for Acquiescent Response Set in Scale Development," The Rand Corporation, forthcoming.

Zeman, R.J., "Dental Attitudes: Layman and Professional," *Dental Students' Magazine*, pp. 321 ff., February 1969.

Zyzanski, S.J., B.S. Hulka, and J.C. Cassel, "Scale for the Measurement of Satisfaction with Medical Care: Modifications in Content, Format, and Scoring," *Medical Care* 13:611-620, 1974.